Does Your Child
Have a Hidden Disability?

Also by Jill Curtis

Where's Daddy? (1996)
Making and Breaking Families (1998)
Find Your Way Through Divorce (2001)

Does Your Child Have a Hidden Disability?

Jill Curtis

HELP YOURSELF

First published in Great Britain in 2002

The right of Jill Curtis to be identified as the Author of
the Work has been asserted by her in accordance
with the Copyright, Designs and Patents Act 1988.

10 9 8 7 6 5 4 3 2 1

British Library Cataloguing in Publication Data
A record for this book is available from the British Library

ISBN 0 340 78679 5

Typeset by Avon Dataset Ltd, Bidford-on-Avon, Warks

Printed and bound in Great Britain by
Bookmarque

Hodder & Stoughton
A Division of Hodder Headline Ltd
338 Euston Road
London NW1 3BH
www.madaboutbooks.com

For John
with love

'The joys of parents are secret, and so are their griefs and fears.'

Francis Bacon, *Essays*

Contents

Contents

Self-help checklists

Acknowledgements

Above all I am grateful to the many parents who were willing to tell me of the struggles they have endured on behalf of their children and to those who were prepared to share their triumphs with me. Also, my special thanks and admiration to the children who know what it is like to live with a hidden disability.

I would also like to acknowledge help from: The National Autistic Society, whose officers read the manuscript and made many useful suggestions; Jane Colby, Chief Advisor from the Tymes Trust, who read the chapter on ME; 'Tosy' from Tourette Syndrome Support for her useful comments about this syndrome; Professor Elizabeth Newson, of the Early Years Diagnostic Centre, for helping me with my understanding of PDA; and Ann Wilson for her wise comments about Dyslexia. Jan Seaborne, Pat Blake, Ann Hicks, Joanna Burgess, my daughters Virginia Ellis and Joanna Hardman and my eldest granddaughter Georgina Ellis all contributed their time and expertise. To them and to so many others, I am deeply indebted, although any faults or omissions are entirely my own responsibility.

My editor, Judith Longman, was as always a source of encouragement and enthusiasm.

Introduction

Don't start worrying dear. Look at it this way. You know when you get a
starter-motor jammed? Seems serious at the time but put it back in second
gear and rock the whole shoot back and forth, she's soon right as rain.
(Peter Nichols, *A Day in the Death of Joe Egg*)

This book is for the large number of parents who find themselves
worrying about whether there is something *not* right with their
child, and perhaps find it difficult to pinpoint just what is wrong
and where to look for help. When do you know if the situation is
serious enough to warrant seeking professional advice? Parents are
often afraid of what might be diagnosed if they investigate further.
If a diagnosis is reached, is the help needed on offer? What if a
parent disagrees with the diagnosis or the treatment prescribed?
What are the overall implications of a hidden handicap not just for
the child, but also for the parents and the rest of the family?

'Invisible' disabilities are among the most distressing of all childhood problems. The range of these 'hidden' disorders is wide, and
overlapping symptoms can confuse even the 'experts'. Therefore, to
add to a parent's worries, conflicting advice may be given.

Once I began the interviews for this book I soon became
embroiled in the discussions of where one hidden disability ended

and another began, and whether some of the symptoms meant a recognized handicap at all. What if you are told, 'He'll catch up',* 'You are an over-anxious parent', or, 'It's his *attitude* you should worry about' – all comments reported to me by parents who suspected something might be wrong with their child? All pointed to the importance of an informed diagnosis, so often surprisingly difficult to find.

Although the nature of the handicap may not be understood at first, the symptoms which *are* visible are most distressing to both parent and child; and these concerns are likely to be shared by relations, friends and professionals, in fact anyone involved with a child with such a disability. The weight carried by the parents is immense, although this is not always recognized. Exhausted parents become frantic in an effort to find help and cope with the day-to-day problems. And often, as parents come to terms with the family crisis, in a desperate attempt to blame *somebody* for what is happening, the marriage itself may be in jeopardy. Parents can become distressed and confused as their child begins to show features which are hard to understand. The signs are not always there from birth, and so can be overlooked in the early days by all but the most in-tune parents. On the other hand, it is important to keep in mind that children develop both emotionally and physically at very different rates. Children's temperaments vary and if your child is at odds with you, or with your idea of what he or she should be like, don't jump too quickly to the conclusion that the child has a disability.

Few children like to be seen, for whatever reason, as different from their peers. And what is valued in one family, may not be in another. For example, one family may be concerned about their child's perceived hyperactivity, but another may see this behaviour as just high spirited. What may be quite acceptable conduct in one

---

*Throughout the text I customarily refer to a child with special needs as 'he' because more boys are diagnosed with invisible disabilities than girls. But, it should be remembered that in practically every case I could just as well have written 'she' and my comments apply equally to girls.

school, may be considered as unruly in another. One mainstream primary school teacher told me that she thought that too many schools expected their children to behave like robots. If they did not conform, then the temptation was to label them as 'problem children with ADD or ADHD'.

It is agonizing for a parent to have to accept that their child has a condition which may mean that now, or in the future, he or she will be disadvantaged. It is understandable that loving parents may hope against hope that the anxiety niggling away at the back of their minds is totally unfounded and that their child will 'grow out of it'. Often they cannot bring themselves to express their fears in words and share their concerns with anyone else, maybe even with each other. This can have disastrous consequences for family relationships. If the disability is great, there is grief at not being able to be the parent you wanted to become, especially if you are constantly challenged by unruly behaviour or night after night of broken sleep.

Some parents told me that with hindsight they realize they fought against acknowledging that there was a problem, since they felt this was a way of accepting a disability in a passive way. Although it may be quite unconscious, this attitude makes some parents reluctant to face up to the situation from the start. The result is to put off seeking help or guidance in the mistaken hope that 'there is nothing wrong'. Those parents who acknowledged early on that there was a cause for concern felt that they and their child had a head start in looking for the help needed. However, getting advice is not always straightforward, and parents are often uncertain about where to turn for guidance. As we shall see, there are serious failings in the help which is on offer. Moreover, there are *still* many doctors, teachers, psychologists and other professionals who dismiss the evidence put in front of them. This lack of recognition is only one of the hurdles parents have to overcome. Parents are concerned that lack of resources is often a factor. Perhaps, after all, we are not living in the caring society we all like to think we are part of.

There are many conditions which affect children, each of which generates its own problems and its own particular requirements for care and treatment. But there are a number of common difficulties and issues which all parents share, and how to gather the right information is one of them. The parents of a child with an invisible disability are likely to be overcome by the situation, and completely at sea about where to turn for assistance and support. A feeling of utter loneliness can be crippling. The pressures on the family of a child with an invisible disability are immense. It is the stress these create, and the devastating constraints they produce, which are discussed in this book.

So what are the hidden disabilities? The most common are ADD (Attention Deficit Disorder), ADHD (Attention Deficit Hyper-activity Disorder), AAP (Auditory Attention Problems), PDA (Pathological Demand Avoidance Syndrome), Asperger Syndrome, Autism Spectrum Disorder, Dyspraxia, Dyslexia, ME (Myalgic Encephalomyelitis or Post-viral Syndrome), Depression, Allergies, Learning Difficulties, Left-handedness, and Speech and Language Problems. However, many disabilities do not fall neatly into a precise category, and even a name given to a disorder such as 'autism' can mean different things to different people.

This book will help you find your way through the maze of conflicting advice and recommendations. Parents who have already 'been there' were very willing to share their experiences of caring for a child with special needs. Parents in the midst of trying to find the best way forward wanted to express their views about the confusion and difficulties they continually come up against.

I hope this book will go some way towards creating a greater awareness of the struggles those children and adults battling with an invisible disability have to face every day of their lives. I have learnt so much from the children themselves and from the parents and carers who support them. Sadly, I have learned, too, that we, as a society, have our own 'invisible' disability: too often we look the other way and close our eyes to the battles, heartache and plain hard work which are there if you are a parent of a child with special needs.

This book is not written from a medical standpoint, but instead focuses on the social and emotional impact of these disabilities on the whole family. I have worked with families all of my professional life, and have become more and more aware of the pressures, largely unspoken, on the families of a child with special needs. First, I listened to the parents, carers, teachers and the children themselves, and then added my own voice to write *Does Your Child Have a Hidden Disability?* These are the words of one of the mothers who contributed to this book:

People need to realize that whatever the outcome, the parents with kids like this try really hard. If anything I say would make just one person feel better that would be good to know.

Part One

Invisible Disabilities

1

A baby is born

We can't form our children on our own concepts; we must take them and love them as God gives them to us.

(Goethe, *Hermann and Dorothea*)

The new arrival

The birth of a baby is usually a time of celebration for the new parents and their families. This joyous moment is the beginning of the process of watching an infant develop in a way which seems miraculous.

When asked whether they want the baby to be a boy or girl, the most common response from both parents and grandparents is, 'It doesn't matter so long as the child is healthy.' If the traditional storybook fairy godmother appeared ready to grant three wishes, the one uppermost in the parents' minds would be for good physical and emotional health for the child in the future.

Everyone who has looked into the eyes of a newborn baby, perhaps only minutes after it has been born, knows the magic of that experience. For the mother and father it is a time to dream of the future for their child. Even the most laid-back parents will allow themselves to indulge in a little fantasy about what their son or daughter will be like in five, ten or twenty years time.

The national screening standards in the UK for mothers and babies improve all the time. For example, every baby born in Scotland from April 2002 will be screened at birth for cystic fibrosis. The Government's pre-election promise is that all babies born in the UK will be screened at birth by 2004. Until recently through failure of a diagnosis many children who were born deaf were not detected for many months, and consequently quickly fell behind their peer group in language development. The NHS are piloting a scheme starting in 2002 called UNHS (universal neonatal hearing screening) which will mean that all babies will eventually be tested for deafness within twenty-four hours of being born.

Once the baby gets the all-clear from the paediatrician, then the parents can relax – a little – and begin the monumental task of getting to know their baby. Parents who before the birth believed they were ready for the responsibilities of parenthood often find to their astonishment they had not anticipated the overwhelming emotion of love and protection they feel for this tiny new person.

Men and women who may have been secretly scornful of friends and relations who boasted about their children's achievements, find themselves bewitched by the cleverness of *their* baby when he learns to roll over on his own or even to smile!

Little by little this new member of the family becomes entwined into our hearts, and all parents know the fear which grips them at the first sneeze or sniffle. But as the baby grows in strength and size the normal anxieties about cot deaths and other dangers begin to recede, and in this busy world the routines of everyday life absorb our attention and energy.

Is there something wrong?

Many parents find it hard to remember just when the thought crept into their minds that there was something not quite right with their child. What often kicks in at this point is complete denial that something is happening – or not happening – in the way it should. The suspicion that maybe, just maybe, there is something to worry about can seem so awful that it is like tempting fate, and courting bad luck, to put into words the anxiety which is making itself felt.

Denial that there is anything to worry about is a very natural instant response to the fear that there is something too awful to contemplate. Believe me when I say that parents need time and support to come to grips with the possibility that their child has a disability.

On the other hand, some parents disclosed to me that they knew very early on something was wrong. Irene said her baby would wake up on an average seven times a night, and rarely had naps during the day. He would cry nearly all the time, and as he was Irene's second child she knew this was not right. The health visitor was concerned about the baby; however, as there was a lot of stress in the family because of the illness of Irene's husband, it was thought the baby was somehow reacting to the atmosphere. Irene said that she knew 'deep down' there was something seriously wrong and suspected the child might be autistic, but like so many parents she did not know enough and was too scared to ask. The health visitor enquired several times if she needed help, but Irene refused because she believed she should be able to cope. Meanwhile, Kevin started to crawl really fast, and at eleven months was running around. He also became an expert climber. Although this brought some envy and amusement from her friends, Irene began to be more certain that something was wrong.

Carrie told me that when her mother-in-law asked her if she was worried about the way that Jenny seemed to be daydreaming all the time, she felt quite ill with shock and replied sharply that nothing was wrong. However, later she began to take notice of something which she had only been vaguely aware of up until then.

A father contacted me to talk about the difficulties he had run up against. His 2-year-old toddler, who seemed to be bright and who hit all his developmental stages, suddenly began to act in a very different way. Little Nigel would not keep eye contact and began to stop using the few words he had learnt. The father said he was so frightened by the change in his little boy that he started to blame his wife and to ask her what she had done to him. This, of course, caused enormous friction between them. Eventually they consulted a doctor who suggested there might be hearing problems and that grommets should be inserted. (Grommets are tiny plastic tubes that are inserted into the eardrum. The fluid which has collected in the middle ear is drained away and allows the air to circulate.) This was done, but with no improvement. In fact Nigel's behaviour became more worrying. It took another year before Nigel was diagnosed as autistic, meanwhile the marriage collapsed. 'We needed help earlier, much earlier. Tell other parents not to "wait and see" and if they have any worries get their child seen by the best.'

Other mothers told me of their early unease when it seemed that they were the only ones to be concerned about a particular aspect of their child's development or behaviour. This was often most notice-able when they were with a group of other young mothers and toddlers. For the hard-to-pacify baby the finger of blame often points towards the mother. For inexperienced new parents it is all too easy to fall into the trap of thinking that it is *their* fault that their baby won't settle. Laurie told me that only when her son was twenty months old did the health visitor agree that something was wrong with this screaming baby; even then no other help was forthcoming and Laurie was still left with the belief that it was her poor mothering skills which were to blame. Looking back, Laurie feels that blaming herself was in fact a way of denying that there was something seriously wrong with her baby. 'I knew there was something up from day one.' It is only now, when her son is seven years old, that a condition called 'pathological demand avoidance syndrome' has been diagnosed.

Cause for concern

Lucy told me that the first sign that there was cause for concern was when her daughter Alice went for her eight-month check and it was noticed that she was not sitting up. 'I hadn't been worried until then.' But it wasn't really until Alice was unable to crawl at thirteen months that Lucy and Tom began to be really distressed. They were referred by a very supportive health visitor to the community paediatrician, who said Alice was in the range of normal. He reassured them that there was no obvious physical problem. Lucy felt that all the professionals she saw were vague about what Alice's problems might be. 'No one seems to know anything. All we can do is wait.' Alice is now being assessed in her new reception class, and although the school say they know she will need extra help Lucy feels she is in a no-man's land and does not know where to turn for more information. All Lucy feels she can do is observe; she notices that Alice constantly walks into things, cannot hop and finds her manipulative control is poor with objects like beads and jigsaw pieces. This is the kind of tension which so many families talked to me about: the on-going, not-knowing state of affairs.

Lizzie told me that it was her husband who first raised concern about their second child. She herself had not been worried because although Maddie did not pass the early milestones at the age her other daughter did, she was confidant in her belief that all children are different and find their own pace. Lizzie's experience highlights the situation for so many parents – is there something to worry about or not? Am I being over-anxious?

Sarah said that she knew instinctively almost from her son's birth that there was a problem. He was 'all over the place' and as a toddler had to be isolated from the other children. But Sarah had to 'fight and scream' every step of the way to get a diagnosis and help. She went through the National Health Service and also tried the private sector. She felt that because she was a middle-class mother there was prejudice against her and she very quickly became labelled pushy and over-ambitious.

A young mother contacted me to say she *knows* that something is wrong with her little boy but not what it is, or how to find help. She feels that his behaviour is too extreme to be normal. She can't take him out shopping as he will not stay in his buggy and at home he raises 'merry hell' all the time. But, she says no one takes any notice of her – except to criticize her. Replying to a letter I had sent to a newspaper about children with invisible disabilities, she was desperate when she contacted me. So what is she to do? She feels that because she is a young single mother on her own she has already been pigeon-holed as a bad mother. She holds that although nobody will take her worries seriously the disturbing symptoms she has to witness are anything but invisible.

'You tell people that what is so terrible is *not* knowing. We've been going round in circles for two years. Everyone telling us something different. Months go by without appointments.' This from a father who is despairing about finding out what is not right with his little boy.

Another father told me that although the professionals they consulted have told him that his little boy has autism there are times when Chris shows signs of being an ordinary child. There are flashes of behaviour which make the family think there is no problem at all, and then their hopes are dashed when he shows other, more worrying signs.

Ella said she knew from his first year that her son was 'different, but I couldn't put my finger on it. At nursery they agreed he "didn't seem right, but not to worry". There was a lot of "See how he gets on", so we let time go by.'

For a child to be handicapped in any way is a dreadful thing. Life is hard enough without the added disadvantage of a physical or mental disability. Parents who are told at the time of the baby's birth or shortly afterwards that their child has an abnormality face a traumatic time. As does the whole family when they have to face the fact that a baby has a birth defect. It would be a very hard-hearted person who did not feel sympathy and commiseration when confronted by a child with Down syndrome, spina bifida, cleft lip or palate or another physical disability which is apparent to even the most unobservant person. A child who is blind or wheelchair-bound is viewed, quite rightly, with sympathy. Not so for a child who may be struggling with depression, chronic fatigue or fighting to maintain self-control over unruly behaviour, or really striving to read or write. If a child has an invisible disability, the story, and the reaction of others, can be very different indeed. You may already have come up against a lack of compassion for a child with a hidden handicap.

Causes for concern
- Take seriously your own feelings of unease about your baby.
- You find your baby is very hard to pacify.
- Your child is late in passing the milestones other children reach.
- He is a seriously overactive toddler.
- Take notice when friends or family express their worries.

Remember, trust your own instincts. You know best!

What are invisible disabilities?

Invisible disabilities can best be summed up as those which are not immediately apparent to the casual observer. A child may be affected with a disability but will not look disabled, and this can be both an advantage and a disadvantage. The symptoms of these disorders are often highly visible, although not always understood, and the symptoms frequently fall into more than one category. Also, more and more new syndromes are being identified, and this can confuse both parents and 'experts'. For parents who ask, 'What causes this disability?' the answer may still be very slow in coming. Sometimes you will be told what does *not* cause it – poor mothering, environment, psychological factors etc. – but the precise cause is often not clear.

Here, to help the reader when the different difficulties which parents run up against are discussed in later chapters, is a checklist with brief descriptions of some of the most common conditions. But, you must remember that for each of these conditions there is a wide band of symptoms, varying from mild to severe. Remember, too, that arguments still rage over whether some of these conditions do constitute a disability at all!

Some of the names used for a number of the disabilities are very similar and the acronyms made from the initials of the disorders get very confusing; you might even feel you are reading a book about codes! Some readers may prefer at this stage to skip these descriptions (up to page 21) and refer back to them later on (they are listed here in the order of the chapters which deal with them in this book):

ADHD (Attention Deficit Hyperactivity Disorder or Hyperkinetic Disorder)

Some professionals maintain there are definite biological reasons to explain this impulsive and restless behaviour and that ADHD is a genetically based neurological disorder, although there are still some who are not at all convinced about this. There is no physical test which can be carried out to verify that a child has this condition. However, what is often believed to signal this diagnosis is an inability to be still, difficulty with concentration, failing to finish what is started, not listening, being easily distracted, acting before thinking, shifting from one activity to another, general fidgeting, anxiety and chaotic behaviour. Children previously labelled as rude, difficult and troublemakers are now more likely to be diagnosed as having ADHD. A child may not necessarily show signs of poor concentration or attention deficit. Many ADHD children also show some of the characteristics of *dyslexia* and/or *dyspraxia* and obsessive behaviour. It is a diagnosis which can only be made by a child psychiatrist or paediatrician.

Autism (Autistic Spectrum Disorder)

This is often used as a term to cover many different syndromes of varying disability. The cause is obscure and as yet there is no test for autism. Researchers believe it is caused by varying factors, including biochemical, hereditary and certain structural differences in the brain. It is seen as a developmental disability which often results in someone having severe problems with communication. There is still much speculation about the final trigger which tips the balance resulting in autism. Autism disrupts the development of social relationships and behaviour. A child may avoid all eye contact with others, have a fascination for spinning objects, insist on adhering to a routine, be very good at rote memory, flap hands or rock, and tend to repeat sounds and dislike playing with other children. Autism may also occur alongside hyperactivity, and the spectrum of disabilities and intellectual functioning is wide, ranging from a very high IQ to a degree of mental retardation. Some children may have a very sophisticated range of language in areas which interest them, others may have poor verbal communication and may speak in a high-pitched voice, or in a robot-like way. For an accurate diagnosis of autism there must be evidence that a child has problems in three areas: communication, social interaction and imagination. Some autistic features may be noticeable without the full diagnosis of autism being given. Some psychiatrists prefer the term 'communication disorder'. Autism can occur on its own, or with other developmental disorders such as a learning disability.

Asperger Syndrome

This is a neurobiological disorder named after a Viennese physician, Dr Hans Asperger, who published a paper in the 1940s describing children who had normal intelligence and language development, but who exhibited autistic-like behaviour and delays in social and communication skills. There is disagreement among professionals about whether this syndrome is part of the autistic spectrum or a separate disability. Children with AS have difficulty with social communication, finding it hard to understand when someone is joking, and an inability to read other people's body language. Being clumsy, disliking change and often speaking in a strange pedantic robotic way are features usually present. Often there is average or above average intelligence and superior language skills. Because children with AS see the world very differently from others, they are inclined to be seen as 'strange' or 'different' from their peers. A symptom which is often present is for the child to be totally absorbed in a narrow interest to the exclusion of other activities. Some professionals will diagnose AS as part of the autistic spectrum (high-functioning autism), others will describe AS as a non-verbal learning disability or pervasive developmental disorder. An earlier diagnosis of autism may be changed to Asperger syndrome as a child gets older and has progressed along the autistic continuum.

ADD (Attention Deficit Disorder)

This tends to run in families. Although some psychiatrists believe that ADD has a biological root, no proof exists of a definite abnormality. As yet, there are no blood tests or brain scans to confirm this condition. Children described as having ADD are easily distracted, have poor concentration and working memory, are forgetful, disorganized, show impulsive behaviour, do not appear to hear instructions and have an impaired sense of time. A child may be easily frustrated, and has difficulty in anticipating events or consequences. This is a condition which can go un-noticed because a child may *be* quiet and so not create problems for others. However, his difficulty in sustaining attention can result in unexpected poor academic achievement and this combined with not listening when spoken to directly may result in him being called careless or naughty.

Auditory Attention Problem or Auditory Processing Disorder or CAPD (Central Auditory Processing Disorder)

This is a general attention problem. A child will have normal hearing but because these children cannot distinguish what it is important to listen to, they are troubled by background noises, affected by distracting stimuli and have difficulty in concentrating.

PDA (Pathological Demand Avoidance Syndrome)

This is a pervasive developmental disorder (PDD) and is related to, but separate from, the autistic spectrum (autism and Asperger syndrome) because children are to all intents and purposes seen as socially skilled. Yet children with PDA are socially manipulative with people and only superficially socially skilled, and they too suffer with social, communication and imagination difficulties. They have extremely good eye contact and use this to manipulate others. They do not have instinctual knowledge of how to play, but will watch and maybe model their own behaviour accordingly. They can be overbearing, clumsy and want everything done on their terms and to their rules. They obsessively avoid demands in a pathological manner and may hit out if restrictions are being placed on them. It is their inability to cope with stress and anxiety which makes them behave in this way. PDA is only now being officially recognized and until recently a child with PDA would have been diagnosed as having 'atypical autism', 'atypical Asperger syndrome' or 'pervasive developmental disorder not otherwise specified'. The difference between the management of a child with PDA and a child with Asperger syndrome is very significant.

Dyspraxia (also known as Developmental Co-ordination Disorder, Motor Learning Problems and Minimal Brain Dysfunction)

This is believed to be an imbalance of the brain resulting in messages not being properly transmitted to the body. Dyspraxic children have no neurological abnormality to explain their condition. Signs are clumsiness, poor posture and balance, confusion about which hand to use, problems throwing or catching a ball, sensitivity to touch, reading and writing difficulties, inability to hop or skip or ride a bike, slowness in learning to dress or feed themselves, a tendency to be impatient. Children are often verbally very adept but may have poor social skills. At the same time they may have inferior reading skills and an inability to express themselves. Although diagnosed as dyspraxic a child may be of average or above average intelligence, but behaviourally immature. A child may improve in some areas with growing maturity and appropriate help and support.

Dyslexia (Specific Learning Difficulties)

There is a clear biological basis to dyslexia. A child who is dyslexic will struggle with reading and writing – letters are jumbled or reversed – there are problems knowing left from right (cross-lateral), clumsiness with lack of co-ordination and poor sense of direction. There are often sleep difficulties, especially in settling at night. Dyslexia tends to run in families.

SEN (Special Educational Needs) or LD (Learning Difficulties)

Children with special educational needs have learning differences which make it much harder for them to keep up with other children of the same age. The cause is often an inability of the brain to process information correctly and in some cases the body is unable to respond appropriately to orders from the brain. This term includes a wide range of difficulties – emotional, behavioural, problems with speech and language, and failure of social interaction. In the UK pupils with SEN are a significant and growing part of the main-stream school population.

Depression

There is not always an obvious reason why someone becomes depressed. Often a number of factors combine together to have this result. Very young children may show signs of distress which need to be decoded and these may include problems with eating, inability to be comforted, being tearful, and problems with sleep. School-age children may refuse to go to school, find it hard to concentrate, and lose interest in play. For older children it is important to consider whether an adolescent is simply uncommunicative or depressed.

ME (Myalgic Encephalomyelitis) or Chronic Fatigue Syndrome or Post-Viral Fatigue Syndrome

The main symptoms are persistent physical and mental fatigue which is severe and disabling, muscle and/or joint pains, headaches, poor concentration, sleep problems. Fatigue is increased by everyday activities. The cause is still unclear, but can be triggered by a viral illness, psycho-social stresses, depression, or can just 'happen'. There seems to be no single cause. Strides have been made with rehabilitation rather than an instant cure.

TS (Tourette Syndrome)

This is a neurological disorder which is characterized by a facial tic and multiple symptoms of movements and sounds often repeated over and over again. Genetic studies show that TS is inherited as a dominant gene that causes varying symptoms in different family members. At present no neurological testing exists to diagnose TS. A lack of fine motor skills may bring problems with handwriting, dressing and tying shoelaces. Obsessive compulsive and ritualistic behaviour is usually present. (The symptom of shouting obscene words, which the media always focuses on, is found in only a small minority of people with TS.) In addition, many children with TS have ADHD and sleep disorders.

As you will have gathered, there are overlapping symptoms for many disorders, and developmental disabilities share many of the same characteristics. A child with CAPD may be misdiagnosed as ADD or ADHD. There is considerable overlap between dyslexia, dyspraxia and ADHD and each can occur with a differing degree of severity. Every child diagnosed as ADD is different, but they will, however, share some of the same symptoms. Dyslexia is the visual or phono-logical processing disorder or a mixture of the two, and CAPD is the verbal (auditory) processing disorder. As you can understand, a diagnosis for any of these conditions requires a sensitive and experienced specialist or clinician who will observe the child very carefully and then follow internationally recognized criteria for a diagnosis. A child who may show signs of autism in early childhood may later develop some basic skills in language within the normal range, and the diagnosis changed to high-functioning autism or Asperger syndrome. In some countries the term Asperger syndrome has still to be accepted, just one example of the complexity of diagnosing many disorders.

Each child is unique

The gradual nagging concern that something is wrong may take some time to absorb, but you should remember that each child is unique. So, you need keep a flexible mind when watching your child, even though the signs which are now worrying you were not there at birth.

Some children can concentrate from an early age, while others are easily distracted. It is unfortunate therefore that parents today are under such pressure. Looking even further back, when I was at school we took in our stride that some of us were good at games or English or maths, and that others had different abilities. We may have groaned a bit when someone we knew who was a poor reader had to read aloud to the class, but that was as far as it went. I may have been at the top end of the class list for literature and history, but I knew full well that I would be very near the bottom for any grading of maths. I can't remember being worried about it, but then as a class we were not assessed and categorized in the way that pupils, teachers and schools are in the twenty-first century. I wonder if today I would be seen as needing special help? Could we really have been more tolerant then than present-day children, teachers and parents are? And was that a good thing? There were some girls who found it easy to be outgoing and to make friends. There were also some quieter, painfully shy girls, but I don't believe that any of us thought they had a disability.

However, that way of thinking seems to have gone out of the window, though it is not necessarily always for the best. Today's children have to show they are up to the mark all round, and woe betide any child – or parent – who does not conform. Look at any group of children of the same age and you will see they are each growing physically at a different rate. It can be hard to be the tallest in a class, and it is not easy for the children who do not grow as fast as their peers. Being 'different' in any way brings heartache to many children, and although size may not be a real issue or concern for your child, it is as well to be careful about how you deal with these growing spurts, or pauses. Comments made even in jest can affect how a child comes to view him- or herself. 'My, aren't you big', or, 'Come on, room for a tiddler' are words which can burn away at a child's self-esteem; they are as hurtful as pointing a finger at a child who is a poor speller or who cannot sit still.

What is it which makes us want to believe that every child can achieve full marks all the time? Does it make us feel 'better parents', or is it that we fear that in this competitive age there will be no place for our child if he cannot learn his tables, or keep up with his Kumon maths homework at the age of seven? Does the child who is quiet, who in earlier times would have been described as 'wool-gathering', have a disability? Some parents may be heartened to know that Sir Magdi Yacoub, the world's foremost heart surgeon has said, 'I forget the names of people, but the science I remember.' He also claimed that as a boy he would sometimes go for days without speaking to anyone. Yacoub recalls that he was much bigger than his peers so people expected more of him. He describes himself as the boy who would sit at the back of the class and say nothing: 'I was too reflective.' What would teachers, or parents, make of him today? So, tread carefully.

'Is it a disability?'

This is a question which will be asked again and again throughout this book. And in many cases it is all too easily answered without sufficient thought, because there are so many disadvantaged children among us. But, for many parents there is also a vast grey area where it is not clear if the symptoms really indicate a problem or not.

Even though your child may show signs of difficulty in one or more areas this may *not* point to a full-blown disability. However, if you suspect that there is something going on which you do not understand, and if the symptoms which are visible are distressing to either you or your child, then this is the time to find out more. It is sometimes easy to convince yourself that a minor blip, which you hope you might be imagining anyway, will not present a problem. And although this is often the case, there comes a time when it is important to explore further even minor concerns.

Sandra told me that she began to worry when her son was seven months old. He was a bit floppy and couldn't hold his head very well. Her GP was supportive and made a referral to the local paediatric clinic. However, all the blood tests came back normal. But she didn't leave it there, and Tom had an MRI scan of his brain (Magnetic Resonance Imaging of the head, the first choice for identifying a brain disorder). This also appeared normal. Even so, she requested a consultation with a neurologist, and the suspicion now is that Tom has a slight abnormality in part of his brain. The stress on the family has been considerable, as they have swung from believing that nothing was wrong, to feeling they needed to pursue more tests. And although they have found the professionals helpful and caring there have been hours and months of waiting around for the next appointment. Sandra said they could see the units were under-resourced, but that, 'This didn't always rush to the front of my mind when sitting for hours in a waiting room, or holding on for months for the next appointment.' It didn't help matters either when an important set of skull x-rays went missing. There was some support during this time from a physio-therapist, and the health visitor was 'wonderful at chasing people for appointments'. But, said Sandra, nothing can prepare a parent for the anguish of waiting to find out whether or not their child has a disability.

It is always agonizing waiting to hear the results of assessments and tests. This is one time when parents need, but often do not get, support from family and from professionals. So learn from Sandra, and try to engage the help of as many people as possible. And keep on going until you are satisfied you have got a full answer to your worries about whether your child has a disability or not.

It is understandable that loving parents may hope against hope that their fears are totally unfounded. Their tentative questions to outsiders may bring reassurance that nothing is wrong, and that they are worrying unnecessarily. This may bring a temporary lifting of the heart, as it is comforting to believe that any suspicion that there is anything wrong is unfounded. For other parents, being prompted to 'Forget it!' or 'Don't make a fuss!' is met by increased feelings of unease.

Perhaps you have turned to your child's grandparents to ask if they are worried about his progress or behaviour. But take care here – today's parents are much more likely to want to know more about 'what's going on' than earlier generations did. Many grandparents will have stories to tell about people they knew as children who were daydreamers, unruly or strange in some way, but who 'grew up all right', and these family memories should not be dismissed out of hand. You may be reminded of a cousin or another relation who is an 'eccentric' or a 'bit of a character' and this may make you doubt that you need have serious worries about your child. One part of you may go along with this, but at the back of your mind the terms 'Asperger syndrome' or 'autism' or 'learning difficulties' may be making themselves heard.

Remember to take into account that although you may have read up on different childhood syndromes your parents or in-laws may not have done. More than one grandparent has disagreed with a diagnosis, calling ADD or ADHD a 'fashionable' name for naughty children. Carol recalled that she violently disagreed with her mother who said she thought that the diagnosis of 'dyslexia' was a soft option for a lazy speller.

Sometimes a parent's fears can send them hurtling down the wrong diagnostic path, so make sure you do not overlook the more obvious solution to your worries. According to the Royal National Institute for the Blind as many as one in five schoolchildren have undetected poor sight. In the UK parents can book a free eye test for their children and it is important that all children should attend on a regular basis. So a baby who avoids bright lights, or a child who has difficulty concentrating, may need help.

'It never occurred to me that my child could have problems *seeing*, it was her disinterest in books which had me worried. Thank God for my health visitor who put us on the right path.' June found that once the problem was detected, the solution could be found. Common conditions such as short and long site, astigmatism, eye muscle co-ordination problems and lazy eyes can easily be treated, and glasses are not always necessary. The RNIB have a very helpful fact sheet for parents.

So, too, with hearing. Children under five can develop glue ear which can cause temporary hearing loss. This may result in delayed speech development in young children and affect a child's behaviour and educational progress. The cause of glue ear is unclear, and boys are affected more than girls. Glue ear (or *'otis media* with effusion') can lead to as much as 50 per cent hearing loss during the crucial nursery and primary school years, and research in New Zealand indicates that children with a history of middle-ear disease display above average hyperactivity and inattentive behaviour.

Professor Tony Wright, Director of the Institute of Laryngology and Otology at the Royal National Throat Nose and Ear Hospital in London, says: 'Studies show that significant hearing loss in young children affects behaviour, the acquisition of skills and speech and language development.'

In the 1970s and 1980s inserting grommets came to be seen as 'fashionable surgery' and a more 'wait-and-see' policy was introduced. The Director of the Medical Research Council's Institute of Hearing Research and Chief Advisor to the charity Defeating Deafness believes the pendulum has swung too far the other way, and children are being denied the help they need. Children become tired and frustrated, lack concentration and do not respond when spoken to. If you are concerned, make an appointment for your child to see your doctor, and if glue ear is diagnosed the first treatment is likely to be an antibiotic. If you are still concerned then ask for a referral to an ear, nose and throat department. You may also want to contact the National Deaf Children's Society helpline for further advice.

So, here is the maze to negotiate: first a decision has to be made about whether the signs are severe enough to need help, and then there is the problem that so many of the symptoms overlap and apply to several conditions. Also, as the disabilities I am discussing in this book are *hidden*, with a wide range of symptoms on a rising scale of severity, it may be some considerable time before anyone acknowledges that a child who is having problems handling everyday situations has a disability, let alone is able to give a name to it.

Is it a disability if your child . . .
. . . does not concentrate
. . . does not conform to 'rules'
. . . does not want to play with other kids
. . . does not spell correctly
. . . does not read
. . . has a sleep problem

. . . is poorly co-ordinated
. . . has a speech problem
. . . has a behaviour problem
. . . is a poor communicator
. . . is disorganized
. . . dislikes change

. . . or is it not?

2

Asking questions

Questions are never indiscreet. Answers sometimes are.
(Oscar Wilde)

'What's *wrong* with you?'

These words have been shouted in frustration and anger at many
children, often by the most loving parents, like when a child does
not fasten a seat belt as swiftly as others. It is painful for parents to
recall how, before they knew that something was really awry, they
thought their child was just being perverse or plain contrary. A child
who is always knocking things over is likely to be called 'clumsy' or
worse, and told a hundred times to be more careful. A child who
can take for ever to get dressed for school in the morning may be
shrieked at to 'Get a move on!' Which parent, if he or she is honest,
has not been exasperated by a child who doesn't catch on in the way
other children seem to? Have you ever told your child to snap to
and not make such a drama out of everything?

This is one of the grey areas mentioned earlier, since it is always
a very trying time when it is not yet certain if there is a real problem.
Does *this* behaviour signal a disability or doesn't it? Each family has

its own pace of doing things. So, for one child always to be late, to have one shoe missing or to ignore some precise instructions can upset the equilibrium. There are other parents who are more at ease with a child's differences, and may be unwilling to accept that he has a disability. If for instance he is always slow to dress, or if he needs that extra bit of help in the morning.

Most of us are used to dealing with several things at once. The radio is on, we are watching the toast, we are pouring milk, and at the same time reminding someone to be home early. To be a child who can only deal with one thing at a time means that he is always in trouble with someone. 'Get out of the *way*.' 'Hurry *up*.' 'Aren't you ready *yet*?' 'Even the *baby* can do that!' Having an auditory attention problem means that you cannot concentrate on more than one thing at a time. Think for a moment what it must be like to be the child: listening to instructions from your mum means that the second sock is not put on. Even the cacophony of ordinary household sounds can be so disorientating that getting dressed for school becomes a daily nightmare. Parents with other younger children who see them getting more organized each day are bewildered. Questions like, 'Why can't you be more like your brother?' 'What's wrong with you?' 'Will *you* get dressed?' slip out all too easily. The child has to pay a high price for having a *hidden* disability. Think how differently a child with an obvious physical problem would be helped to prepare for the day.

It must be terrible to be bombarded constantly by sounds and signs which are incomprehensible. A child must feel like an outsider living in a strange land, a place where everybody else seems to know the rules. If you realize that on top of this some hidden disorders make it impossible to distinguish between different emotions, you will have some idea of what it must be like to be a child with an unrecognized disability.

You will hear from the children themselves in a later chapter, but here I want to mention Helen who told me that she has suffered all her life from ADD (attention deficit disorder). When she was a child she wondered why grown-ups always seemed to be shouting at her. Only years later did she realize that her parents and her teachers after calling her once, twice or even more times would raise their voices to get her attention. She wished she had understood that when she was growing up because as a result she became frightened and developed into a timid little girl.

The parent/child anxiety spiral

What must it be like to have ADD or ADHD *before* anyone realizes there is a problem? 'Sit *still.*' 'Why can't you concentrate like anyone else?' 'For goodness sake, pay attention.' 'I have told you *that* a hundred times!' These are only some of the things said to these children. Indeed, parents reported that as the symptoms become more obvious and intrusive, they cannot help getting more and more exasperated and exploding with angry outbursts at their children. This is, of course, brought on by a mother or father's uncertainty about what is happening and what to do for the best when 'ordinary' parental strategies don't seem to be working. This in turn adds to the anxiety of the child, and the spiral can escalate with alarming speed.

Brenda and Gordon told me that they were at a loss to understand just what was troubling their 8-year-old daughter, Ruth. There were times when she just 'wasn't there' and all the shouting in the world didn't get her to respond immediately. They thought at first she might have a hearing problem, but after her hearing was tested and found to be quite within the range of normal, they didn't have a clue where to turn to next. Is it a disability if a child just 'shuts down' at times? Is it a problem if a child appears to daydream to such an extent that others begin to notice? Is it an emotional, neurological or other problem? Is it that she is just a quiet, reflective little girl who has a lot of imagination and likes to be off in her head making up stories? Does this child have an invisible disability?

Many parents are devastated when they remember how they dealt with their child's behaviour before they could accept that there was a hidden handicap. These symptoms can, and do, cause social as well as educational problems. But, keep in mind that parents are human and somewhere inside themselves they shy away from accepting that their child is struggling. It is preferable to believe that the child is careless or lazy and with a bit more effort could do the hundred and one things we ask our kids to do.

Audrey told me that two of her nine grandchildren have problems of some sort. She was unclear about the nature of them, but they surfaced in appalling behaviour and the kids always succeeded in upsetting any family occasion. She felt unable to deal with these boys, and swung between encouraging her son to find some help for them while shouting aggressively at them herself. 'I knew it was a spontaneous reaction, but unfortunately I couldn't hold it in when they lashed out at one of the younger children, or kicked the cat.' Audrey felt at her wits' end because she could not decide whether there was a problem, or if they were just very unruly boys who seemed to be getting away with murder. She told me she had 'cried and cried' with worry but seemed to get no nearer to finding out if her grandsons needed help, and if so, what kind?

Children who are dyslexic may be quite clumsy and often take a tumble. A health visitor who noticed the many bruises on Daisy began to have worries about child abuse. She persuaded the mother to take the child to the clinic for a fuller assessment and it was then that other difficulties were diagnosed. This gives cause for thought about the outcome if help had not been at hand.

Parents can easily lose confidence that they are doing the right thing by constantly correcting a child's behaviour. Or, to take the example of a slow reader, is it helpful to make time each day for a reading lesson? If the session ends in tears (not necessarily the child's but the mother's, as has often been reported to me) the answer is probably not. However, it is very hard for caring parents to stand back and not have one more go at spelling or reading, in a final effort to help their child to overcome his difficulties.

Katie told me that her son Henry would not sit still long enough to learn to read, and the school told her she had to make him read every evening. It caused endless problems and rows between them. When he would, or could, concentrate for a moment or two he picked it up very quickly, but getting him to settle was the problem. Katie said she regrets the pressure it put on them both which for a while affected their relationship. 'Because he is bright, it took a long, long time for him to be diagnosed as having ADHD.'

Andrea told me that her eldest two simply picked up reading skills almost over night, and it puzzled and annoyed her that Liam didn't catch on in the same way. 'I know I ended up screaming at him when he seemed to gaze around the room instead of getting on with it.' Andrea also admits that she felt quite frightened when she began to see that the carefully chosen books meant nothing to her son. 'I bitterly regret those times I yelled at him. I couldn't believe that he just couldn't remember words like "the", "that", "can" and "would".' It was also the time when she felt a chill around her heart and began to wonder if difficulties with reading and writing were the forerunners of a wider area of concern.

Other people may ask why 'Ronnie' always breaks things, or why he won't play, or you overhear other children teasing or questioning him about why he is not able to read or write his name. If you started off shouting 'What's wrong with you?' in anger and end up thinking to yourself the more fearful 'What *is* wrong with my lovely child?' things have been brought to a head and must be tackled.

Teasing and bullying

A child who is a victim of bullying is often a child who is different in some way, so this may be a sign that he has a hidden disability. Some children can all too easily become victims of harassment and humiliation. Sadly, at a very early age this teasing may set up a pattern to haunt a child throughout his school life. If a child has a tag affixed to him – as 'difficult' or 'demanding' or 'the child who can never remember to be in the right place at the right time' – he will begin to see himself in these terms. Consider for a moment how we behave towards a child who is friendly, proficient in class or at sport and who constantly receives a large share of praise. This child will eventually carry with him an aura of success and confidence. Sadly the reverse is true, and the child who is slow on the uptake, who cannot grasp some concepts and has poor motor or social skills soon sends out a negative message, which in turn gets reinforced by others.

We can all remember how sarcastic teachers used to get cheap laughs out of the class at the expense of the less successful pupils: 'Last *again* Rupert, who would have thought it!' 'Paint spilt, don't tell me – let me guess, Ruthie did it!' 'I want someone to read out this notice to the class – no, not you Jamie, I want it read to the class *this week*!' Or, 'Wake up Patti, off with the fairies again?'

Children with a learning disability can be very sensitive when this is happening to them. A child who is autistic or who has Asperger syndrome may to some extent be protected from the digs and the mocking which can go on; some simply do not notice as they are absorbed in their own world. But many children with a degree of learning difficulties are only too aware that others are laughing at them even though they are, for example, unable to grasp a mathematical concept.

This is where some children become expert at covering up, or masking their disability in the best way they can. This may take the form of an attitude of 'I couldn't care less' or some other form of self defence, but all the while the joking is whittling away their self-confidence, so that, as well as a learning difficulty, they come to have very low self-esteem. Once this sets in, it is difficult to shift. The child who cannot learn to read begins to despair, and if in addition he or she is not able to keep up, say, at sport it may mean the child will become expert at avoiding awkward situations. This will affect his or her social interaction, and adds to the picture of the child being 'different'.

Another result of being bullied is to become a bully oneself, so if your child suddenly becomes more aggressive and his behaviour deteriorates check this out. Again, the press made much out of the story of an 11-year-old boy who was expelled on his first day at secondary school. His mother was reported as saying , 'He is easily provoked . . . it is because of being bullied that we taught him to stand up for himself.' This little boy had earlier been excluded from his primary school.

Children with Asperger syndrome are especially likely to fall foul of bullying. It is as if they have no way of defending themselves against the 'teasing' which takes place. I don't much care for the word 'teasing' in this context, since for me teasing has an element of affection in it. What I am talking about is verbal or physical intimidation; a child who cannot distinguish between what is bullying and what is a joke is in for a hard time at school. To be told, 'You are over-reacting' – which is what many children probably are doing – or, 'Sort it out yourself' is going to confuse a child with Asperger syndrome, as he tries to decode what seems to him a foreign language.

Just think what it must be like to lack the social skills and ability to deflect bullying. What to you or to me would be the rough and tumble of the playground becomes a setting for abuse and cruelty. No child should be left to deal with this on his own, and it is an insensitive parent or teacher who tells a child, 'That's life', or, 'Don't bother me with it.' So, you should take any signs your child is being bullied very seriously, and if he is unlikely to tell you about it, watch for any bruises or unexplained marks on his body. Be on the alert too if your child begins to behave differently for no apparent reason, such as not wanting to go to school, slipping behind in school work, mislaying some prize possession or money, or any other 'out of character' signs. These may all point to the child being harassed or tormented at school or on his daily journey there. If your child's behaviour suddenly changes dramatically, bullying may be a reason for this.

A child with Asperger syndrome, who takes practically every remark literally, may be picked upon and 'set up' by other children. Such a child will do as he is instructed by the other kids, and as a result may not be able to tell who is a genuine friend. He may even be egged on to steal or damage property. When the sky falls in and the teacher appears it is the child with Asperger syndrome who will say, 'Yes, I did it', while the other kids will keep quiet. I have heard of this happening from parents in many different places.

So, if your child has any of the signs we are considering, keep a close eye on the behaviour of other children. They can often home in on a child who cannot control his temper. Knowing that to goad such a child will bring on a furious reaction frequently makes it a popular sport. So, if your child is involved in more than the normal number of playground fights, make sure the teachers are aware of this. If your child is already at nursery or school, make sure you have investigated their anti-bullying policy. Be certain your child knows the procedure for talking to an adult about any bullying which is going on. In the UK, kudos is now attached to schools calling themselves 'telling' schools; this means they encourage children who feel they are being harassed or bullied in any way to speak to specially designated trained pupils. The knowledge that it is okay to speak up is an important one, because a child may be under threat of repercussions from the bullies if they talk to a teacher or parent. Being armed with the facts will enable your child to feel safer and capable of doing something about it, knowing that he will be believed and supported.

If you suspect your child is being bullied – or if your child has told you that this is happening – take it very seriously indeed. Changing schools will not be enough. Two schoolgirls in the UK, who were victims of bullying, killed themselves within a few weeks of each other. In both cases they had each told their parents what was happening, and the parents had then asked the school concerned for help. When the bullying continued the parents moved their daughters to new schools. However, the girls were still victimized as in each case the perpetrators lived near by. One girl had been singled out for being 'different' because she was very tall for her age, the other because the media had reported her donation of bone marrow to her sister who was suffering from cancer. The suicides of these two young girls highlights the importance of protecting our children right up to the hilt if there is any hint of bullying going on.

Children who have played together for some time often show great kindness and understanding to a less able child. If there is a handicapped child in your group you may have found it is a wonderful way for children to learn about compassion, and about helping those who need assistance (unlike the attitude of those who drove the bone marrow donor to suicide!). It is often later, when meeting up with new children, that 'teasing', or worse, can come about.

A first-class site on the Internet is Bullying Online (www. bullying.co.uk). Parents, children and teachers will find support and practical information on this site.

Be on the alert for bullying
- A child with special needs is particularly at risk of being bullied.
- 'Jokes' and 'sarcasm' can whittle away at a child's self-esteem.
- Take action if you notice your child becoming more aggressive.
- Your child suddenly doesn't want to go to school.
- Your child 'mislays' some prize possessions.
- Your child gets into more fights than usual.
- Your child has torn clothes or unexplained bruises.

The time to look for help?

It is a major decision whether or not to ask for help. There is only one guideline: *when a parent thinks it is necessary*. If a parent is sufficiently worried to want an outside opinion, then this is the time to seek professional help. When a parent finds his child's behaviour becoming more bizarre or difficult each day then this is the moment he needs to have confidence in his own feelings and judgment to fend off friends and family who tell him not to fret. 'All children are different.' 'He's a dreamer.' 'She needs handling differently.' 'You give in to him.' 'Why do you have to make a problem out of everything?' 'She'll learn to read in her own time.' '*Make* him concentrate, *I* would.' 'Be tougher.' 'Be softer.' 'Your expectations are too high.' And even the blunt question: 'What's wrong with him anyway?'

I was told of instances where total strangers would say, 'Can't your son control his temper? If it was *my* child . . .' These are the kind of remarks many parents have to face. In fact, several parents pinpointed the moment they decided to look for help was when they realized that the family could no longer give any advice which was effective.

It is worth remembering how you used to feel about children whose behaviour betrayed signs which at the time you didn't understand. Corrie said: 'I recall with deep humiliation that before my son was diagnosed as autistic, I really didn't care about mentally disabled people. I saw them as a burden.'

Where to go for assistance

Once it is decided to look for professional help, the next hurdle is where to ask for assistance.

Maxine screwed up all her courage to go to her GP and ask for help for her boy who was literally climbing up the wall at home and at school. When Maxine suggested that he might have ADHD and be in need of help, this was rejected out of hand. 'Don't waste my time! Get your husband to control him if you can't,' was the reply. Familiar to you?

Unfortunately, that GP was not alone in dismissing a worried parent. What is so cruel and shows an unthinking attitude is that even if the doctor will not go along with the ADHD suggestion, no other help is suggested or offered. There are psychologists and psychiatrists who think like this too. All too often parents are told bluntly that it is the upbringing which is the worry, and one mother who eventually read her child's medical file was appalled to see a memo saying, 'This mother has Munchausen Syndrome By Proxy' (MSBP is a condition whereby an individual makes another person sick in order to look for medical help and intervention). This child was later diagnosed with pathological demand avoidance syndrome.

Parents like Maxine, who are looking for help for their child, may all too often find themselves referred for marital counselling, which of course adds to their sense of failure at a time when they need all their strength. Carrie told me how she felt ill with shock when told that she had been referred. Her immediate reaction was, 'I came here thinking I was a failure as a mother, and now they think I am a failure as a wife.'

Annie finally persuaded her husband to go with her to the family centre to ask if there were any strategies they could use to help their son. His behaviour was causing major problems. They were horrified to be told that the only help on offer was for them to see a social worker weekly for six weeks in order to assess *their* relationship. 'They didn't even ask to see our son Andrew.'

Of course, as a psychotherapist I know that there are situations in which a child picks up conflicts within the family, and – in social work terms – 'acts out'. If there has been a bereavement in the family, a breakup, or even the birth of a new baby a child may respond by out-of-character behaviour. Naturally children can become stressed, too, by events outside the family. But, to assume from the start that it all stems from problems in the parents' relationship to each other does not help anyone. I urge professionals to work more sensitively with parents who are already distressed enough about having to seek help. More casework is now family-based, and this is to be welcomed, but what this entails needs to be explained in detail in order to enlist the co-operation of the parents; it must not be assumed that they are the enemy. To inform a professional couple that they need to 'see a social worker' without talking through the policy of the unit is harsh, especially at a time when feelings are raw. I know that when they get this reaction from a clinic it can, and does, frequently cause untold damage. Especially if the parents are, at this stage, hoping that some simple concrete strategies will help put everything back into place. In many cases it results in a family withdrawing from outside intervention.

Deb asked for help at her daughter's school when she had become sick with worry about Nancy's behaviour and her manner of communicating with people. The school said she was 'moody' and a 'drama queen' and 'immature'. The head claimed Nancy set herself up for the bullying she endured. At seven years old! She was doing well academically, so the school were not worried. Deb left the meeting feeling even more at a loss about what to do next. Parents desperately need back-up and support to underpin their feelings and instincts if they are worried about their child's development and have to brace themselves to confront the 'experts'. The most common reaction from a professional, usually the GP, is 'Wait and see'. All very well, but this can leave parents feeling that *they* are the ones who have the problem and are making an unnecessary fuss! It can also mean that precious time is lost. 'Our doctor told me that our son is autistic and we should more or less accept it and get on with it. That was all the help we got.'

One mother, Molly, told me that she first felt that 'things were not right' when her son was one year old. 'Something' inside her made her feel that the way Alan behaved was adrift, although it was hard to put her finger on exactly what was worrying her. Time went by, and a visit to her doctor brought an insensitive reprimand with, 'You have a boy, and boys are like this.'

As the months went on Alan's behaviour caused more and more anxiety. Again and again Molly was told that she was making a fuss about nothing, yet every day Alan became harder and harder to manage. Friends and family became less supportive and as no babysitter could manage him, Molly felt she was trapped with a child who was out of control. Yet still the family doctor would not take Molly's worries seriously, and adopted a jostling-her-out-of-the-situation tone. Many of the characteristics which were causing trouble for her son were apparent to Molly in her husband, and she is convinced that if Bill had grown up in today's climate he would have been diagnosed as having ADHD. Her mother-in-law backs this up with numerous stories about Bill's childhood.

Because father and son are in many ways so alike it brings about head-on collisions and there are terrible rows and even physical fights. Neither of them will ever wait a moment for something they want, and when they are both at home in a small flat their surplus of energy is hard to contain. Molly said her husband was not overly worried about Alan's behaviour, and at times Molly wondered if their difference in views about parenting strategies added to the stress shown by Alan. A few months after talking with Molly she contacted me again, to say that Ritalin has now been prescribed for her husband, but not at present for her son.

Sally, too, told me she knew there was a problem with her son from very early on, but again visits to the doctor only brought criticism, and pep talks about how boys will be boys. This meant that Sally began to blame herself for her poor parenting skills and over the years her confidence as a mother plummeted to zero. Sally and her husband Rob even went to classes in parenting skills and saw a marriage counsellor and, eventually, Sally asked her doctor for some antidepressants for herself. 'I was literally banging my head against the wall. I didn't know what to do. I took the tablets, but I am not depressed – I just don't know what to do!'

Meanwhile her son continued to cause chaos, and no childminder would look after him. Even the grandparents, while 'loving him to bits', found him too unruly to look after. But, at the same time, they told Sally and Rob to stop worrying, and 'He'd be fine'. 'We knew he was anything but fine,' said Sally, but nobody would listen to us or offer help in any way. Fortunately, Sally has a friend who is a psychologist and she arranged a private appointment with a child psychologist who right away diagnosed ADHD. Having been dismissed by their doctor, health visitor and paediatrician the relief was colossal, but this soon faded into anger when they realized that they had had to pay for this consultation with money they could ill afford.

Sally said she hoped I was spelling out clearly just what looking after a child who has ADHD is like. 'It's not just overexcited, you know.'

When Irene saw her GP and voiced her worries she was told her son would calm down once he got to school. Irene knew she could not wait that long. The health visitor suggested that Kevin might be hyperactive, and although a search in the library proved fruitless, Irene did find out about the Hyperactivity Children's Support Group (see page 246), and she became convinced that diet was something to be sorted out.

Maddie said she knew there was something different about her baby when he was just a few months old. He was very active, but would not communicate with her when she wanted to play or talk to him. On the other hand, it seemed as if when he wanted to make contact with her he could and would succeed in doing so. He stood at six months, and when he crawled he crawled at the speed of light. He didn't walk, instead one day he just started running, and would run all over the house. Sometimes Maddie felt he ran to get away from her. At two years old he was trying to beat up his older sister, and at three she could not contain him. The GP spoke of ADHD, but when Derek was prescribed Ritalin he turned into a zombie; when the medication was changed to an antidepressant his behaviour improved for a while until it seemed to become ineffective. Different specialists said different things: 'atypical autism' and a query over the diagnosis 'ADHD'. 'So back to square one,' said Maddie. It took two more years, and a terrible fight on her part, before pathological demand avoidance was diagnosed.

On the other hand Pamela told me that when she was worried about the language development of her son she took him to the GP, who immediately referred him to a speech therapist. The speech therapist's opinion was that the boy needed more help at school and so at four years old Bill was 'statemented'. (A 'statement' is a confidential and legal document relating to the educational needs of an individual child. In order for a statement to be produced, a child must be proved to have special educational needs which require special educational provision.) However, this was not as advantageous as Pamela hoped, and during the next two years when Bill was at nursery school he received no extra help. 'Nothing,' said Pamela, 'no help at all.'

Amy told me that there is nothing worse for a mother than when no one will listen when she tells them that her child has a problem and needs help. For years Amy fought – 'And I mean *fought*' – with the school, the educational psychologist and the doctors. They all told her that her son was very bright, but lazy. Amy said she knew something more than this was wrong, but because Sammy had a high IQ he was dismissed as a difficult and awkward child. His report would say 'Sloppy work', 'Very careless', 'Work spoilt by inattention to detail'. Amy went into battle, even to the extent of contacting her Member of Parliament, and because she made such a fuss she became labelled as a very troublesome parent. This caused a rift between Amy and her husband, and very nearly broke the marriage.

Only when Sammy got to university was dyslexia diagnosed almost right away. His tutor could not believe that Sammy had not been diagnosed at an earlier stage in his education. Sammy now has a PhD, and Amy wanted me to include her story – her crusade – in the hope that it would encourage other parents who are seeking help for their children to challenge the objections they come up against. She says although she did fight, she wishes that she had fought even harder for her boy. 'Just think of those years he struggled *without* any help, and he was so unhappy at school. And all the worrying and arguments very nearly broke up our family.' Amy offers a sense of hope to any parent and child who get bogged down in the tangle of unsympathetic professionals. To keep on going when there was no chink of light anywhere was the hardest thing to do, but together Amy and Sammy did it.

Parents will often hesitate because they are not sure whether they are looking at a disability or just a delay in maturation. 'Or is it *us*?' is a question many of them ask each other. And on top of this the difficulty in getting a diagnosis often means there is unnecessary delay in getting appropriate help for a child. But this should not be allowed to happen.

The true situation, which can leave a bitter taste in a parent's mouth, must be faced, since only when it can be accepted that their child is in some way disadvantaged or handicapped can helping their child truly begin. Remember, saying the name of a disability will not make the condition worse; and *not* saying the name will not make it go away.

Use this check list to decide when to look for help

- It is the parents who know when it is time to look for help.
- Don't get confused by the different advice which will be offered by friends and family – listen to your own voice.
- Professionals should listen to a family's concerns and take them seriously.
- If your first port of call for help does not bring results, don't give up. Prepare yourself for a fight.
- Start near to home – consult health visitors, nursery carers, teachers and your family doctor.
- 'Mother knows best', so don't be cowed even if some guidance is still needed about whether there is a problem or not.
- Don't be afraid to ask questions.

3

Getting a diagnosis

A physician cannot cure a disease, but he can change its mode of expression.
(Thomas Hardy)

The importance of a diagnosis

There are families who struggle for years to get a diagnosis and this may not always be because there is a lack of professional help on offer. They may be reluctant to press for more information in the hope that the signs they are aware of do *not* mean their child is in any way disadvantaged. To be fair, some professionals are reluctant to give a clear diagnosis right at the start, even if they could. The reason for this is that giving a name to a child's disorder can act as an indelible label, which remains with the child for the rest of his or her life.

Another reason is that a dual- or multi-diagnosis is often necessary because so many symptoms overlap as the line between different disabilities is blurred. Dyslexia, dyspraxia and ADHD are three disorders which frequently show duplication of symptoms, often with different degrees of severity. Because there is such a wide spectrum of similar symptoms it may mean that a child is diagnosed with one disorder to the neglect of another, with the result that there would be little room to manoeuvre in diagnosis or management.

As we will see in more detail in a later chapter, a child with symptoms which point to dyslexia may be referred to an educational psychologist, while a child showing fairly similar symptoms may be judged to be dyspraxic and be referred to a physiotherapist or occupational therapist. And yet another professional may feel the same signs point to ADHD and send the youngster to a child psychiatrist. These different diagnoses can on occasion be prejudiced by the belief that one diagnosis, for some extraneous reason, will be more 'acceptable' to the parents than another. Some professionals are probably right in feeling that a final diagnosis should only be given if it then provides a clear route towards help for that individual child.

A caution came from Barbara, who urges parents not to get a diagnosis 'simply for the sake of a diagnosis'. Her own experience was that when she asked for help from a local assessment centre she was told that her son did not have ADHD as they had feared, but that 'he simply had an attachment disorder'. End of story – for the professionals – but not for Barbara and her family. Barbara, who had no idea what this really meant or how best to help her son, was left more confused than ever about how to treat Billy with his ever increasingly disturbed behaviour. I was shocked to hear that this experience is more common than we like to believe. Even if a diagnosis is obtained there may be little or no follow-up. So, how useful is it for a parent to be handed some such comment, but then left, literally, to hold the baby. Or, as in Barbara's case, a 7-year-old who could not be left for a moment, had terrible mood swings and who had been excluded from school?

When Annie's daughter was diagnosed with bipolar disorder (manic depression) she had known for some time that this was on the cards. Annie had recognized many of the symptoms from other members of her family, so she was already prepared to accept that her daughter had a lifelong disability. What she decided was that she wanted to appreciate *this* child *now*, and work with her daughter's strengths. Annie believes very firmly that the family needs to 'surrender' and accept, so as to get right behind the child with the disability. Many other parents echoed this and urged every parent of a child with special needs to get in tune with the child as he *is*, and not always to be wishing and hoping for more.

However, there can be comfort and relief in getting a 'name' put to the disability. Many parents told me they felt it took some of the responsibility off their shoulders. Janice: 'Oh the relief. Right! My son has ADHD, now we can get cracking to get the right help.' Janice had suffered badly from criticism from both her family and complete strangers about her son's behaviour in public when he appeared to be out of control. Now that she had a diagnosis she felt she could silence her critics, and that she had something to use as a weapon to get the help her son needed. Janice was able to explain to other parents too about her son's condition. She was encouraged to find that as a result they became much more sympathetic and supportive. Whereas she had been left in lonely isolation waiting outside the school, now she was included in the mothers' chat, and some went further and asked if they could help in some way. Luke, her son, was even invited out to play after school, and she also felt that in time it would help him to have an explanation of why his behaviour was so out of order. 'For us, the label was the key we needed to open the door for a lot of support and understanding.'

However, there is often heartache once it is out in the open and it is confirmed that a child has a disability. Also, what is a parent to do if they disagree with the diagnosis? It can take courage to ask for a second opinion. But, one of the most substantial things a parent can do for a child is to ask questions, and to go on asking questions. You have to be a voice for your child, and it has to be loud, clear and strong. Pauline bitterly told me, 'You have a better chance of being heard if you have money.' We will explore this avenue later in another chapter.

Jennie told me that after searching and searching for help her son was diagnosed as having ADHD. She found it hard to accept, but then made it her daily task to find out everything she could about the possible cause and the ways she could help her child. 'I played it by the book.' The shock came three years later, when a new consultant dismissed the diagnosis and said that Wills had an auditory attention problem. Jennie wept with frustration when she talked to me; she could not start from scratch again. What problems had this misdiagnosis meant for Wills?

Pros and cons of getting a diagnosis
- Some professionals are reluctant to jump too soon to a conclusion, since they believe that to give a quick diagnosis may mean a child gets labelled incorrectly.
- A dual- or multi-diagnosis confuses the issue for some time afterwards.
- A firm diagnosis can help you to get the help your child needs.
- A diagnosis may remove the anxiety and uncertainty for parents.
- It can be easier to explain the situation more clearly to other people.
- People may be more sympathetic to a disability which has a label.
- There can be heartache when it is confirmed that a child does have a disability.

Keeping records

You must ask any professional who sees your child for a written report, so that you can gradually assemble a full picture of your child's strengths and the areas where there is cause for concern. You should keep a record of the clinic or health centre, the consultant's name, the date you visited him or her, and the outcome of any contact you have had with every organization or professional. And you should take the time to make a few notes of the conclusions reached; this will help you to get clear in your own mind what was said. You may need to refer to these records again and again over the years. Parents I saw in my research for this book often had a file brimming with information they had gathered over the years. A record of the routes already taken can save time and energy, and prevent getting caught in an endless loop of referrals.

Generally, you should gather as much information as you can about your child's development and keep detailed notes about the milestones he has reached, especially in relation to his peers. If you are unclear about anything, ask the professionals you are in touch with for a fuller explanation and for any guidelines about how you can help your child. Don't be put off by medical terms, or an explanation which does not make sense to you. Speak up if the professionals start to talk in jargon; many of them are guilty of doing just this. Pauline told me that all she wanted to know was why her daughter did not talk when she was at school, but she had to listen to people discussing problems about 'fine motor responses to stimuli' and other equally unfathomable terms to the layperson to describe the behaviour of her child. Although she was well educated and articulate, she was totally baffled by a report sent to her after one assessment which was full of medical terms.

Be on the lookout if anything is referred to simply by initials. After a consultation Pam found herself with her child outside the consulting room door, and could only recall that she had been told her daughter 'obviously had SLD'. Don't let this happen to you. Pam could only discover by telephoning a friend who was a social worker that SLD stands for 'severe learning difficulties'. I am sure the consultant didn't deliberately confuse her, but as in all professions the experts think everybody is as familiar with the shorthand terms as they are themselves.

It is also a good idea to take somebody else with you if you are seeing a consultant. Otherwise you may find that watching your child, trying to explain the things you want the consultant to know, plus trying to listen to what is being discussed is rather overwhelming. If you have another adult with you she can take over looking after or distracting your child, leaving you free to do the talking and listening or making notes about what is being said so that later you can have a really clear account of what was discussed.

> *Getting the best out of a consultation with a professional*
> - If you have some idea about what you think is wrong, get as fully informed as you can in advance. Draw up a list of questions in advance.
> - Make sure that being given a diagnosis does not mean the end of help on offer.
> - If you don't understand what you are being told, say so!
> - If you disagree with a diagnosis, ask for a second opinion. It is your right.
> - Keep notes of all contact with outside agencies.
> - Ask any professional who sees your child to give you a written report.
> - Take someone with you who can care for your child, so that you can see the professional alone if necessary.
> - Send any letters by recorded delivery or hand deliver them.
> - Find out as much as you can about the condition. Search the library, Internet and get in touch with any organization specific to the problem.

Fight, fight and fight again!

Every parent who spoke to me said that anyone who needs to find help for their child must be prepared to be tough and forceful. Sandie said it went against her nature to be too direct and she always tried to keep a reasonable tone of voice, but she learnt to say what she had to say. 'If you don't, you will get the run around.'

You should always keep in mind that you know your child better than any 'expert', so if you are uneasy about any aspect of your child's development or behaviour you must speak out. If *you* don't make a fuss, nobody else will. It quickly became evident to me how even the mildest parents had to get the bit between their teeth to fight for what they believed their child needed. Pamela, who helped me a great deal with this book, said the most important message to convey to parents is that as soon as they suspect that their child may have special needs, they must be prepared to fight for assistance every step of the way. 'Never stop,' said Pamela, 'and never give up.'

'Keep badgering them,' was also Pauline's advice when she described how she had to phone time and again to get an appointment. She also said that a parent can easily get side-tracked by the professionals when they concentrate on one thing at the expense of another. She had not thought there was any problem with her daughter, a shy little 3½-year-old. But at a routine check-up she was told bluntly, 'There is something wrong with your child' and the search to find out *what*, began. She became frantic to learn why her little girl was mute at school, but would talk at home. The professionals she was referred to were more concerned about the discrepancy between the child's verbal skills and her comprehension. Pauline's priority was to understand why her daughter was not speaking outside the home. 'Don't be distracted by the professionals – go for what you think is the problem.'

Pauline and her husband had no idea at the beginning just how many people from different professions they would see. 'We saw community paediatricians, educational psychologists, speech and language therapists, an ophthalmologist, a music therapist, people from the sensory integration unit, occupational therapists, consultant paediatricians, and I think there were more.' She told me that every one of them seemed to say something different, and although she could accept that her daughter's condition needed to be diagnosed, she found the experts' attitudes very conflicting and sometimes confrontational. She was told within a short space of time that her daughter had 'selective mutism', 'dyspraxia', 'dyslexia', 'hearing problems' and a 'mild expressive language disorder'.

What were Pauline and her husband to think? 'This is where the fighting had to come in. They wanted her to have grommets (we said "no"), play with a bean bag twice a week (we said "yes"), listen to special music through headphones (we said "yes" for a while), therapy for mutism (too much pressure on her and she became very stressed), but we also had to plough through different diagnoses.'

As their daughter is a graceful little girl they would not accept the diagnosis of dyspraxia; as her reading was okay they would not accept dyslexia. As they felt it was a speech problem they opted for speech therapy only to find there was a one-year waiting list in the National Health Service in their area. As their daughter was by now six years old, they felt time was of the essence and so they found a private speech therapist to work with Betsy. They have settled on the diagnosis 'subtle dyspraxia' and are hopeful that with the help of the therapist there is every chance that she will catch up with her peers in a social sense. 'They are discovering things all the time, and I believe there is a hope that her brain can correct itself before the age of ten.' They are aware how fortunate they are to be able to pay for a private speech therapist.

'Fight? I'll say so! We had one run-in after another,' Claudia told me. Her daughter could only speak a few unconnected words at the age of four, so she tried everywhere to get help. She was told, 'You live in a bilingual household, what do you expect?' and 'Maureen is the youngest of four, the others do the talking for her.' They were made to feel over-anxious, fussy parents who were exacerbating the problem by taking their daughter for assessments. As soon as they went to an educational psychologist, again privately, they at last found a diagnosis and the help Maureen needed. Claudia: 'I would hate to think what would happen to a kid whose parents accepted those early rebuffs, or who could not afford to pay for some help.'

Parents who disagreed with the diagnosis or treatment, usually found they had a dispute on their hands with the professionals. Pamela: 'When I finally got my son to be seen by a paediatrician, he wrote down, "Marked autistic tendencies" and I objected immediately. Admittedly Bill has communication difficulties and this is one of the autistic traits, but there is a big, big difference between just some of the traits and having full-blown autism. The consultant agreed with me in the end, but they should be more careful.' Of course, not all parents come up against these problems, but from all the accounts I know of, a battle was the norm.

What's in a name?

Professionals can often be very heavy handed when talking to parents about their children. 'We were given a report to read at the end of the meeting, and I read it on the bus. It said George was autistic, so we heard just like that. No one had mentioned the term before.' From another parent: 'Your child has learning difficulties and will never achieve the high standards your family expects. With those words we were shown the door. My husband and I looked at each other with horror. We weren't given a phone number, an appointment, or any offer of help or support at all.'

I also heard from Sue who said that as a young single mum she was told by everyone she spoke to that it was her fault for not being able to cope with a young boy. Indeed, the prejudice she came up against as a mother on her own made it impossible for her to go on looking for support. 'I had no fight left in me.' Years down the line she is battling with guilt over the fact that she then kept quiet about her worries and did not look for the help her son needed. But who can blame Sue who said that at eighteen years old with an overactive toddler all the fingers pointed to her inability to 'bring him up properly'.

Bess saw a consultant whom she thought was assessing her son Richard for a tonsils' operation. In fact she discovered later that she was a child psychiatrist. 'This doctor sat there and said Richard has ADHD.' Bess had never heard of it and when she looked puzzled the doctor gave her a leaflet which has a checklist on it for ADHD. 'He had all those all right – I could have written it. Then we were out of the door. Not a suggestion of where I could get some support for Richard or myself – or really what ADHD is. Just a leaflet.' Richard had always suffered from night terrors and Bess was surprised to see that this was listed as one of the symptoms. She had repeatedly taken him to the doctor over the years because of her concern about his fears and his out-of-hand behaviour, but had always been told to get a grip and tighten up on her parenting. At the time of the diagnosis for ADHD Richard was ten and a half years old.

Another problem I heard about from a number of mothers and fathers was that once their child was diagnosed with a particular disorder, the child seemed to lose his individuality and become the 'ADD child', or the 'dyspraxic little boy'. This is something to be aware of and of which people in general still need to be better informed. How often have we heard a child described in a way which sounds dismissive, such as, 'Well, she has Asperger's'? Labels grouping children into categories do not help them retain their self-esteem as individuals.

Thankfully we have learnt to talk about 'learning difficulties' rather than the old terms of 'mental retardation' or 'mental handicap', terms which had become stigmatized by their use in a pejorative sense. Others could well copy the Down's Syndrome Association's example: they have made sure that the public no longer refer to a child as a 'mongol' but to someone 'who has Down syndrome'. There is room for a lot of improvement if we are to remove totally the element of shame or embarrassment attached to the names of some disorders.

Don't rush into it

There are many parents who feel they were pushed into getting a diagnosis. Today so much is talked about behaviour management that when parents, who are unsure of their parenting skills, are told that their baby sleeps too little (or too much) they believe that there must be something wrong. Even more experienced parents can be thrown off balance, as I have heard from several mothers. They have been advised to allow 'controlled crying' and 'controlled comforting' without the professionals taking sufficiently into account the individual make-up of each and every baby. If something like this is happening to you, follow what your heart and instincts tell you. You and you alone will know if your baby is in distress, and you are the best person to understand what is troubling your baby. If your baby is very small it may be too soon for anyone to pinpoint that something is wrong. So, don't try to rush any professional into a diagnosis because babies and young children can change dramatically in those early months or years. It may be very hard, but take some time to watch and see how your baby develops.

Gather as many observations about your child as you can, so that when you do see someone for an assessment you have all the relevant facts and information to hand. In this way you will be able to give a clear and precise outline of your child's particular symptoms and special needs. This will go a long way to ensuring that you receive the support and services you need if they are available.

The range of hidden disabilities is wide, as you will see when I discuss them in detail later in this book. But, you should also keep in mind that there can be a huge variation in the degree to which a child may be affected by any particular disorder. For example, you may hear that a child has been diagnosed as autistic, but autism covers a wide spectrum of disorders and the degree of their impact in his particular case needs to be evaluated properly. A variety of symptoms confuses not only the parents but frequently the 'experts' as well. As more and more syndromes are identified this also makes getting a diagnosis more complicated. Just think how in the past children with special needs were either referred to as 'spastic', 'retarded', 'backward', 'slow' or ESN (educationally sub-normal). Today no parent would be satisfied by, or accept, these labels and as more sophisticated assessments are developed, a diagnosis can be so much more precise. Unfortunately, since not every professional is experienced with all the disabilities, this is not always so. Therefore, be patient if you are referred from one specialist to another.

False hopes

There are a wide variety of symptoms for many conditions. And although some of these may appear in isolation and can then be attributed to a specific disorder, very often it is not as straightforward as this. It is all too easy to go down the wrong path, therefore it is vitally important not to jump to conclusions too soon.

Some parents have to brace themselves to accept that there is not a precise diagnosis for their child, and this can lead to frustration and fear that without a diagnosis there will be no help on offer. In these circumstances it is as well to steer away from seeking, in desperation, an appointment with one more specialist in the belief that a definite diagnosis will improve the situation. And remember, a diagnosis is not a cure, although it is only too easy to hope that one automatically leads to the other. In an effort to do 'the right thing' for their child some parents do literally go to the ends of the earth to find someone − anyone − who might be able to put their finger on what is wrong with their child and *make him better*.

False hope can be raised by people promising a cure, and while it is totally understandable that a desperate parent will try almost anything, do be on your guard against unrealistic promises, especially if there is a financial outlay involved. Margie told me that when she was at her most desperate to get help for her child with ADHD she saw a notice in the local paper offering help for any child who was hyperactive. What she found was that a vitamin supplement was being sold, and at each meeting parents were expected to pay. 'We just don't have that kind of money,' said Margie.

When well-meaning friends tell you, 'There must be something which can be done,' it somehow implies that you haven't done all you could. It may be impossible for them to believe how hard it is to get help, and they will often think that it is you who have not pursued every avenue. It is as well to prepare a few well-chosen phrases to ward off inquisitive or interfering people. 'Have you tried this − have you tried that?' 'Isn't there some drug you can give her to calm her down?' 'Surely you are not giving him drugs?' are the sort of questions you will be subjected to. Try saying something like, 'I don't want to talk about it now', or, 'We are still trying to understand what is happening.' If said with a smile such ripostes can deflect even the most obtuse friend (or stranger!) from further questioning.

Alice looked for help when her son Ben showed a marked inability to mix with children, as well as having speech problems and learning difficulties. Her doctor began to talk about ADD (attention deficit disorder), but coincidentally at the same time Ben needed surgery for undescended testes. The surgeon was concerned about the development of his scrotum and advised genetic testing to establish the possible cause. The results came back with a diagnosis of an additional x chromosome, a condition which is known as Klinefelter's syndrome (KS, more recently referred to by calling those with the syndrome as 'XXY males'). This is usually only diagnosed in later life, often during adolescence when more obvious physical changes take place or when as adults the sufferers are seeking advice on fertility. Although it may be thought of as a physical disability, children with this syndrome usually learn to speak much later than other children, and may also have difficulty learning to read and write. And most have some degree of difficulty with language throughout their lives, especially of expressing how they feel.

Alice went on to explain how complicated it can be to have a child with an invisible difficulty which no one seems to have heard about. Neither her doctor nor the paediatrician had any experience of caring for a Klinefelter's boy, and not surprisingly none of her friends had any idea what the condition meant. She explained about it to the pre-school and kindergarten which Ben attends, but only because he has a tendency like other KS children to wander. Through her initiative on the Internet Alice has managed to make contact with other parents of KS children and she is comforted and helped by this, especially as she foresees additional difficulties when Ben reaches puberty.

I have spent some time describing Alice's problem to illustrate how complex the situation can be and how important it is to leave no stone unturned. This often requires great patience and perseverance on the part of the parents. Alice believes that the diagnosis came as a mixed blessing but one which prevented her, and Ben, from going down the wrong road.

On the Internet there is one site, http://specialchild.com/diagnosis.html, which many parents contact if they are unable to get a diagnosis. Parents post details of their child's symptoms in the hope that someone else, somewhere, will be able to identify a specific condition.

The long term

Parents can become distressed and frantic when their child begins to show features which are hard to understand. And although, as we have seen, there are many different hidden disabilities which can affect children, whatever they are, the worries which they prompt are the same for all parents.

Moreover, the awful truth is that for some conditions there is less tolerance and understanding from the world at large, than for others. Also, while most families and some friends will rally round for a family crisis or emergency, when a condition is ongoing and requires help day in and day out, some people cease to be supportive or even sympathetic. This is especially so if it is a disability which carries with it disruptive or anti-social behaviour.

Many mothers and fathers told me of the sickening moment when they realized that friends were no longer forthcoming with invitations, and that the most loving relations were reluctant to invite a child with severe behavioural problems. Even mothers who have been part of a toddler circle of young mums found themselves being shunned when the other children began to notice that their child was disrupting their play hours. 'Why doesn't Ben play with the other children?' 'Why doesn't Polly sit quietly at times and listen to a story?' All this adds to the isolation and panic felt by mothers and fathers in those early days when their previously secure nursery world becomes unsafe and unsure.

Parents, coming from all directions and with different concerns about their children, will share varying degrees of disbelief, isolation, grief, guilt, rage and panic. At the same time they all have a plethora of anxieties and aspirations in common. It is to these shared feelings, self-doubts and to the 'frequently asked questions' they pose that we will now turn our attention in finding the best way to face up to the situation.

Order of battle for getting appropriate help for your child
- Never forget you are the real expert on your child.
- If you don't make a fuss nobody else will.
- If you don't understand what you are being told by an expert, ask for an explanation.
- Gather all the facts you can about your child's possible disability.
- Remember that not all the worrying signs necessarily add up to a disability.
- You don't have to account to friends and family for what you are doing.
- Be prepared for a long war, never give up.

4

Facing up to the situation

Well, of course, you find out gradually, not all at once.
But there is a point when you finally accept it.
(Peter Nichols, *A Day in the Death of Joe Egg*)

Is it anyone's fault?

All parents who discover that one of their children has a hidden disability agonize over questions such as: 'Why my child?' 'What has caused this?' 'What shall I do now?' Anger usually follows hard on the heels by asking, 'Who is to blame?' For you feel there must be someone whose error or negligence has brought about this disability. These days parents are inclined to attach blame to a variety of causes – environmental problems, diet, negligence on the part of the medical team when the baby was born, or genetic conditions – although there is very little positive proof either way. Knowledge about genetics has increased by leaps and bounds over the years, and it is now possible to confirm a number of diagnoses – but by no means all – using the different tests available. However, beware of falling into the trap of expending too much energy on trying to apportion blame; you are likely

59

to come up against a brick wall when you are unable to find the cause.

This will misfire as accusations fly through the air, and if self-blame appears to be the only answer then you will be carrying an additional burden along the way. If you get caught in this way of thinking it will be only too easy to find something which you wish you had or had not done during pregnancy or shortly after your baby was born, or perhaps just yesterday. Speaking to as many parents as I did when interviewing for this book I was dismayed to hear how often a note of self-recrimination crept in.

Karen told me that when all the professionals seemed to be unanimous in saying there was nothing wrong with Iain, the only conclusion she could come to was that as a mother she had failed her son. She felt judged by the world at large, and often felt like screaming, 'I am doing my best.'

People – strangers even – can be extraordinarily insensitive with their remarks. I was told of comments such as, 'I bet you smoked during pregnancy, didn't you?' and, 'Fancy you letting him have that MMR injection, haven't you read it causes problems?' It seems that most people feel safer if they can pin the blame at someone's door.

Ways to avoid apportioning blame
- Don't spend your energy trying to find who is to blame. There is unlikely to be a simple answer.
- Knowing the cause is not likely to guide you to the right remedial action.
- You may end up unjustly blaming yourself or your partner, which is not going to help your relationship.
- Don't let anyone else salve his conscience by blaming you.

Is immunization the cause?

As the debate rages on about the wisdom of immunization, parents are left in no-man's land. Almost every day an article appears in the newspapers imploring parents to give their child the MMR vaccination for complete protection against measles, mumps and rubella. Meanwhile the triple vaccine has aroused fear in many parents who suspect that it may be linked to autism and bowel disease, and one British drug company is working on plans to add a fourth vaccine to the triple jab, to treat chickenpox.

One doctor in the UK has offered an alternative to parents by vaccinating children against measles, mumps and rubella with single injections and as a result he was referred for investigation by the General Medical Council and was under threat of being forced to stop practising. Headlines in some newspapers said that he was putting children's lives at risk. However, his appearance before the GMC was eventually dropped because of insufficient evidence, and he was cleared of professional misconduct, a major blow to the Government's attempts to persuade parents to choose the combined MMR jab. Inoculation rates in some parts of the UK have fallen to an all-time low as parents seek advice about the possible dangers of the triple vaccine. Meanwhile, Dr Mansfield believes that he is providing a choice for parents who might have decided not to have their children vaccinated at all.

The disquiet about permitting individual vaccines is the extended period over which the vaccines have to be given, since there must be at least three weeks between them. Although another reason – which I find hard to accept – is the claim that parents will not be motivated to go back for all three vaccines. However, a new GMC ruling now permits a GP to give single doses of the vaccines. (For more information visit the website www.jabs.org.uk.)

Expert opinions are put forward to claim that there is a link between the MMR vaccination and autism, while this is hotly denied by other experts. The latest theory is that it is the mercury in vaccines for babies and infants which has caused the steep rise in cases of autism. Although a link is denied, the Department of

Health in the UK is phasing out the use of mercury-based vaccine for infants, but meanwhile doctors are being instructed to use up old stock, even though the same vaccines are available without mercury. This ruling ignores the advice of the American Institute of Medicine, which is that supplies should be withdrawn. In America the Center for Disease Control and Prevention has agreed that vaccines containing mercury will no longer be used for children.

The European Union has just begun a £2.5m review of the possible adverse effects of the triple vaccine, but the results will not be known for three years. Meanwhile many parents are worrying about it, and if your child is showing signs of autism and he has already had the MMR vaccination, you may use this as a reason to blame yourself. Don't do this. Remember that autism was known and diagnosed long before the MMR vaccine was ever used. Childhood diseases such as measles, mumps and rubella are almost unheard of in Britain now, and you may be too young to remember just how sick children could be with these childhood illnesses.

Meanwhile the debate rages and the buck, as usual, stops with the parents. 'I can pinpoint the day my child changed. I know it was the MMR vaccination. Since then I have read that a child with an antibiotic allergy should not be vaccinated. I didn't know that then. Parents are kept in the dark.'

Equally there are parents who are concerned about a possible link between over-prescribed antibiotics for babies and toddlers, and a later disability. 'I *know* my son was fine until he had a virus and was hospitalized and pumped full of penicillin which they now find he is allergic to.' Alice: 'My son had many ear infections as a baby and was prescribed antibiotics. Now I wonder if it is my fault for letting him have them. I have read that it can cause trouble later? I should have known better.'

It is also true that parents sometimes notice signs around the age of one which may point to autism, and this is about the time of the first injection of MMR. But, you should know that nearly one-third of the children later diagnosed as autistic develop normally to start with and show signs of autism after their first birthday.

A study in Finland concerning the MMR vaccine given to 1.8

million children was funded by the manufacturer; naturally parents are sceptical about the results. So, who is a parent to trust?

In the US, the National Vaccine Information Center will be a help to many parents. The NVIC is a non-profit educational organization founded in 1982. They state: 'Vaccines, immunizations or inoculations are recommended for every child born in the United States. A vaccination shouldn't hurt a child but sometimes they do. Before your child takes the risk, find out what it is.' So, go to www.909shot.com for more information from this Internet site dedicated to the prevention of vaccine injuries through public education.

Don't blame yourself

It is a cruel and unnecessary punishment to blame yourself or *your partner*, but it happens. At a time when parents need to support each other sparks often fly and accusations of 'You don't understand' only add to the pain of the situation. I believe that the furore which can erupt at this time is actually a way of masking pain. It is rather like banging your head against the wall to shut out a deeper hurt, that your child is having to cope one way or another with a disability, *and you don't know how to help him*. The shouting which goes on is one way of drowning out a voice inside which is telling you that there are troubles ahead. Feelings of depression are almost universal at this time too.

One of the cruellest allegations made against parents, usually the mother, is that it is somehow her depression or anxiety which is causing the disability. Not so long ago the media were full of articles about 'refrigerator mothers' – meaning those who are cold and unloving – who were accused of being the cause of many childhood conditions ranging from schizophrenia to autism. But, tell me which mother would not have moments of deep depression or anxiety while trying to find out if a child has a disability or not? And yet there are these charges, and none more hurtful than to be told, '*You* are causing your child's illness, and encouraging her to stay away from school.' Perhaps you find this difficult to believe, and yet Joan, whose daughter suffers from ME (myalgic encephalomelitis), was told just that. This is a dreadful accusation which has been wrongly attached to this very debilitating and terrible illness.

Pauline, the mother of an 8-year-old who was eventually diagnosed with ADHD, told me that she felt so angry at the unfairness of it all, coupled with the injustice she met, that she thought the strain would kill her. She found herself sinking under the pressure of believing that the cause of her son's behaviour was something she had or had not done. After one more sleepless night she decided that the way through for her was to become very active in the field of helping other families cope with a child with this syndrome. 'For me,' said Pauline, 'it was either get so angry I thought I would go up in smoke or educate myself sufficiently to be able to inform others. Luckily I chose the second route. Of course, I had to educate myself first, but we all benefited from that.'

How will you cope?

A question you may be asking yourself is, 'Will I be able to cope with what lies ahead?' Can you pace yourself for what might be a long haul? Perhaps you have never in your worst nightmare considered that having a child would involve 24-hour care, 7 days a week, 365 days a year. Yet, this is what it is like for some families. Of course, the disability which your child has does not mean that every moment must be spent planning and looking for help. But for many families, concern about a child is somewhere in the background *all* of the time. And even the slightest disability may cause traumatic blips at unexpected times.

Children who, for example, need very little sleep can be very hard to care for day after day. The sheer tiredness of parents which accompanies this can wear down the most loving family. 'My boy who has ADHD needs four to five hours sleep max, and that's on a good day.'

A meal out, or a holiday, provides a welcome break for most

families. But if your child finds it difficult to conform with the 'rules' of society, then an outing will be anything but restful or relaxed.

Bob told me that what caused the most difficulties in his family were arguments over trips. 'We were okay at home, but going out with a kid who is likely to cause an uproar is not my idea of a day out.' So what do you do? If you have one child who will either not be able to keep up physically or will most likely bring about a disruption, do you deny the other children in the family their days to the sea, the lakes or theme parks? Many children who are within the autistic-spectrum range do not like being out of their familiar surroundings. They like routine and feel safe and secure at home and, for them, and the family, a holiday can turn into a nightmare. So unfortunately you must take this into account.

The most common cause of grievance from parents often surfaces around what to do or not to do: 'Nobody told us anything.' Alex had no idea of the stress his 7-year-old son with autism would experience when the family went on holiday to France. Indeed, the little boy was so unhappy and so obviously distressed that the family had to return home. Only when little Henry was surrounded again by his familiar objects would he settle. 'We would never have done it', said Alex, 'if we had had any idea that this is a common feature of autism. Why do all parents have to learn by trial and error? You tell parents that from me.'

Audrey told me that it was when her child could no longer be restrained in a buggy that the problems became more noticeable. In the end her husband would go on ahead with their other sons, while Audrey kept at Bobby's pace. Audrey also dates the beginning of the end of her marriage to this time. Tim, and the boys, began to enjoy a life which was denied to Bobby; to compensate for this, Audrey spent more and more time trying to find activities which she could enjoy with her youngest boy.

Laura told me that the day she had been told – rather bluntly – that her child was showing all the signs of being within the autistic spectrum disorder, she read about a mother who jumped to her death with her 11-year-old autistic son in her arms. She said she cried and cried, not only for the mother and child, but for herself and her child. It made her determined to get as much support as she could both for her daughter and for herself. It made her very much aware of the pressure that a parent can feel and she became determined to find a network of support.

What often comes to the fore with surprising speed though is a heightened feeling of protectiveness and care towards your child with special needs. It makes no difference whether your child is an 'only' or you have two, three or more children. Once you realize that you have a vulnerable child it can be only too easy to find that all your attention is going towards that child. Often this is at the expense of the other children in the family. It is a big mistake to think from the start that you, and only you, can care for your child and you alone can understand how to handle him so you must be there at all times. However difficult it is to accept, you must realize this is unfair to the rest of the family, and not in your child's best interest either. Your child will come to believe wrongly that only 'mummy' or 'daddy' will do.

Jenny said that she soon began to accept that she could not cope on her own. Her mother was helpful, but two children with ADHD meant that she was not able to take them both out at the same time. Living in a small flat is a nightmare as she has to use all her energy to keep them quiet and occupied. 'Get help. Get as much support as you can. Speak to other parents with children like this.'

One major problem for parents is when they are given a range of near-impossible tasks by different professionals. You have to do research into all the treatments, you have to find the resources for these treatments, where are they available – remembering to telephone back the person who promised to call you – look for local support groups, learn about different exercises, monitor the child's medication, check food for additives, 'practise this and practise that . . . because *if* you do it right your child should improve'. And of course you have to do all this with broken nights and lack of sleep!

Guidelines for coping with the situation
- Get support anywhere and any way you can.
- If you can't find a network of support, consider setting up a local support group.
- If possible, share the care of your child right from the start.
- Try not to be overwhelmed by everything you have to do.
- Take every opportunity there is for a welcome break – a meal out or short holiday – you deserve it!
- Don't neglect your other children; they need attention too!
- Remember, children with autism and other disabilities like routine.
- Don't subject a child with a hidden disability to anything that is beyond his capabilities; choose suitable activities.

Talking to your partner

It is a sad fact that the pressure of caring for a child with special needs puts great strain on a marriage. At the very time when parents need to pull together it all too often brings about a rift, and the relationship cracks, especially if one parent is taking the main thrust of the care and concern.

The pain of discovering that *your* child is disadvantaged is so horrendous that people choke on the words – even to their nearest and dearest – and I believe that this is the obstruction which so often gets in the way and prevents talking and real communication. One partner's desire not to add to the burden which he knows the other must be feeling prevents many couples from weeping together over the sorrow of what is happening.

The best way to manage a child's disability often causes a disagreement between parents. What appears quite a minor disability to the outside world may not seem like that at all to the family. If one parent believes that a child 'could if he tried' be less of a burden while the other sees that the child is struggling hard to overcome the problem, the inevitable happens and the parents disagree in a heated way which is not helpful for either them or the child.

Most parents want their child to be seen in a favourable light by others, so if your child is beginning to show signs of restlessness or overactivity then prepare yourself for some unwelcome attention when you are out in public or with friends or family. This is an important issue to discuss with your partner. Anthea only discovered after some time that her husband could not cope with the attention which always accompanied an outing with their child. Until she realized this she just felt he had no interest at all in family trips. Once this was in the open they could plan excursions where Charlie could 'run riot' and nobody would comment.

You will have to harden yourself to the looks of disapproval and exasperation which come your way, a very trying thing to cope with. 'I have toughened myself to this. If it gets too bad I say to people who are staring, "It's not your problem and it's not your business." But it hurts.' You will need to brace yourself to accept that things will almost certainly get worse; a 'toddler tantrum' with a 2-year-old is one thing, but when your child is fifteen years old it is quite another. Recently Anthea overheard a passerby say, 'Look at that kid, he must be mental.'

Pam, with two boys diagnosed as ADHD, said she often felt like screaming aloud when out shopping: 'These boys have a disability and we are all doing our best.' She refused just to stay at home with the children, and she found the reaction of other people very painful until she learnt to ignore them; she kept her tears for when she was alone at home. She felt her husband had no idea what it was like for her to go out each day with the children. 'Have you told him?' I asked her. 'Oh, no, it's best I don't give him any more grief.'

There is another good reason for getting a name put to a certain disorder, if possible. Jean told me that only when her husband was told by their GP that the diagnosis the specialist had come up with was dyspraxia, would he finally believe that the different symptoms were not a collection of awkwardness, laziness and just plain bloody-mindedness. Jean said her husband's whole attitude changed, and he became the front-runner in campaigning for extra help for their boy at school. From then on they were as one when dealing with their son's disability.

Keeping in step is very important, so try to make sure one parent does not become the 'expert' while the other is out of touch with day-to-day developments. This way resentment lies, with accusations of 'You don't understand', or, 'I *told* you weeks ago that we had an appointment with the specialist tomorrow.' No matter what, take care of your marriage. As Ali said: 'Don't add a broken family to your child's worries.'

Battles can go on raging long after the breakup of a family. If one parent feels that the way to deal with an obviously very distressed child is medication, and the other parent doesn't, then the battle truly rages. After Penny and Paul divorced, their 10-year-old began to display many of the symptoms associated with a diagnosis of ADHD. Penny believed he could be helped to be calmer with medication, but Paul saw their son's distress as a natural reaction to the family breakup. No other dispute in their divorce caused as much pain as this clash of opinion over the care of their son.

Remember, too, that people show their feelings in different ways. Don't dismiss a partner as 'not caring' because he or she isn't grieving or is not up in arms about the matter in the same way that you are. One person's way to cope with a situation may be very different from another's. One mother told me she couldn't believe her husband could show so little emotion when their child began to have distressing symptoms, with the result that she began to discuss the situation with him less and less. Only years later did she discover in a roundabout way that he suffered a great deal at that time too but was unable to express his feelings; he kept them tucked away inside himself. Sadly, over time his feelings of loss and grief were converted into a depressive illness.

Don't become so preoccupied with your child that you forget that the rest of the family needs loving care too. Make sure, if you can, that you have grandparents or friends or babysitters who, properly primed, can care for your child for even a short spell so that you can be together as a couple and get refreshed. Make a positive resolution that not every moment of any time off will be spent in talking about your child and what the next step for him is. It may be hard to do but you will feel the benefit.

I realize that at the other end of the scale, for those parents who discuss each and every step, the transitions as a child gets older will be more complex. I will consider later in more detail about how difficulties are likely to multiply, for although most people are tolerant with the behaviour of very small children, this understanding begins to evaporate all too soon. You may already have an inkling of how the gap is widening between your child and his peers, both educationally and socially. This glimpse of the future may cause you heartbreak, although your child may be oblivious of any difficulties at present.

Talking to each other about your fears
- Make sure you *do* talk to each other – and listen!
- Agree on rules and strategies for handling the situation.
- Keep in step about treatment and appointments.
- Make sure any babysitter is carefully primed about your child's condition.
- Always remember people show their grief in different ways.

Telling your child

A debate rages about when and what to tell a child who has a hidden disability. For a parent who cannot bring him- or herself to accept that a child has a difficulty, which not only will not go away but will be more of a handicap in later life, this decision can be a torment. If you cannot bring yourself to say out loud, for example, 'My child is dyslexic, therefore has a real problem with reading and writing,' and instead you blur the issue by saying something like, 'My child isn't interested in books,' then how can you help your child to understand what is happening?

'I am sorry, but I cannot say the "A" word, even to myself.' This kind of comment is more usual than one might believe, and some parents who were very willing to talk to me skirted around using the actual word to describe their child's disability. Audrey said she still felt sick every time she thought of the term Asperger syndrome, and at present there was no way she was prepared to discuss this with her child. She said that she could talk to him about specific difficulties she knew he was having, but 'that word' would seem to her as if she was telling him he had something which could not be mended. A dad in Australia told me that neither he nor his wife would use the word autism, and if driven would refer to something like 'that thing you have' when talking to their child.

If you are having a problem admitting out loud that your child has a disability, why do you think this is? Of course, it is a very painful thing to have to accept that your child is handicapped in any way. It is not only unpalatable for the sake of your child, but it can also hit at your own self-image. It may be quite a narcissistic blow – and a blow which some parents cannot recover from. Ask yourself if the invisible disability has touched within yourself a chord of shame or prejudice?

Judy told me that when she first knew that her son was not developing at anything like the same rate as her other children had done, she felt nothing but deep foreboding. She found that it was quite hard for her to go on caring for her little boy in quite the same loving way. Judy was brave enough to tell me of the bad period she went through. Every time she saw Edward chuckling and smiling something seized her heart. When she saw him struggling to cope with eating or walking, she had to turn away. Her husband noticed this, and it was only after opening her heart to him that she remembered that there had been a child with a disability at her school who had been regularly teased and bullied by the other children. Judy remembered to her horror that at times she had been part of this tormenting gang, and the memory of those days had been activated by watching her son. For Judy, a child who was 'slow' was in for a bad time, and she felt there was a strong element of shame attached to the condition. After Judy had put the pieces into place and seen the whole picture she was sickened by her memories, and only then could she separate them out from her care for Edward. She was then able to talk about the way Edward, unlike her other children, was struggling, and at last she could face up to what might be the problem.

Children are quick to catch on to the fact that their peers, or even younger siblings, are reading fluently, and many a child is left feeling that it is his own fault if he can't. This is especially so if there has been some earlier shouting and anger with exhortations to 'try harder' or 'for goodness sake, I told you what that word is only yesterday!' Some parents try to reassure their child that he will catch up and not to worry. But if you are eight years old and all your friends are reading and learning their tables, this is not very reassuring. Most parents say nothing at all.

In her book *Martian in the Playground* Clare Sainsbury describes what growing up with Asperger syndrome was like for her. 'I alternated between believing that because my experiences and feelings were so different from everyone else's, I must have incipient schizophrenia . . . and convincing myself that, just as everyone kept telling me, there was nothing wrong with me and I could be like everyone else if only I tried harder. (I must not be trying hard enough.) The fear and misery that this caused should be easy to imagine.' I am only too sorry to say, 'Yes, it is!' and to think how hurtful this must have been for Clare. Speaking as she does with the experience of someone who has been on the other side of a disability should make us all pause for thought.

Consider what it must be like always to be last, never to have the right sports equipment, always to be in trouble over *something* and not to know why. Dorrie: 'I was torn between telling my kid that he had a disability and so wasn't to think he was naughty or careless for forgetting everything – and feeling if I did that it would let him off some hook and he would stop trying.' Ron: 'Okay, we got a diagnosis of ADHD, but we also had to draw the line at his anger and behavioural problems. We couldn't ignore them.' Yet, another parent told me: 'If your child was blind you wouldn't go on hoping that one day he would see that there are dangers all around in the street, would you? You would warn him, and explain.' As Gloria said: 'In this world there are disabilities and there are disabilities. Ones that you can't see are the ones which cause problems in the outside world.'

I have been told of parents who have T-shirts with the words 'I am autistic – please be patient' printed on them for very young children to wear. Whenever I have mentioned this, it brings very mixed reactions from other parents. Often, an initial gasp of horror is followed by a more considered approach that it might in fact help the wider public to be more tolerant and more watchful for the safety of a child. A publisher in the UK gives away badges with 'I love someone with autism', 'I love someone with ADHD', or, 'I love someone with Asperger syndrome' on them. One mother who wears the autism badge explained to me that it gets people talking to her on the bus, in shops and outside the school, and in this way she hopes to make more people aware of something which should not be spoken about in hushed tones.

Patti told me that she has had no difficulty in telling her children that they have ADHD. She has explained to them repeatedly that their condition is nothing to be ashamed of. It is something they just have to live with. She wants them to know that medication does not cure their condition, it is a tool to help them. And they have to work hard to use it. She feels that explaining this to them has helped, and they often appeal to her when they need extra support.

Eileen explained that as her family had difficulties in understanding *what* was wrong with Phil, how could he possibly grasp the problem. Once again, we hear of the conflict of a parent who is unable to focus on just what is not right with her child.

A more recent medical attitude has been to involve a child in the discussions. So, you should be ready for this. It will mean that your child will have plenty of questions for you, and if you don't have the answers say so, or tell him that you will find out. In these circumstances you can be sure your child will want to know more about his condition and helping him to understand will enable him in turn to explain things to his peers. Talking together with your child will help you both to put your feelings into words, and you are sure to be surprised to hear what has been going through his mind. The fact that he has learning difficulties does not mean that he is necessarily unaware of the attitude of other people towards him. It will make things easier for him if you can find a way of opening up a discussion.

You may have to struggle together to find the right words. One 11-year-old who talked to me about the difficulties she had been caused by being cross-lateral and judged by others to be exceptionally clumsy and awkward, said: 'Mummy explained to me that some people are good at some things and not at others, and also that people shine brightly at different stages in their lives.' This simple explanation, which had so obviously helped this little girl a great deal, is an example of how the right words at the right time can have an impact upon a child. And, of course, upon the way they see themselves.

The more easily you can talk to your child about his or her hidden disability and the consequences, the more your child will be able to cope. Tell your child that you understand that some things are especially hard for him or her to do, and if possible try to work together to find some strategies or routines which will help. A child who is chaotic and disorganized can be aided by making sure that all school equipment is labelled very clearly and school bags are packed in readiness the night before. If special shoes have to be taken to school on Wednesdays, or a swimsuit on a Friday, then post a sign up in the kitchen to remind you both. A see-through bag will make it easier for you to know at a glance if the right books have been packed for school.

It is not only the child with a hidden disability who has to be told something. Other children in the family will wonder why 'Helen is not able to learn her tables or is slow at reading'. This can be puzzling if Helen is an older sibling. It is kinder to give a brief, age-appropriate explanation.

Carrie told me that she had never discussed with her older daughter the fact that her little brother has any difficulties. What took her breath away was overhearing her daughter, with her arm around her brother, explaining to a shop assistant that he couldn't speak very clearly 'because he has a problem, you know'. She said it brought tears to her eyes to hear this, and she felt badly that she had never thought it necessary to talk to her daughter or to give her any explanation.

Other children can be less supportive of a brother or sister with a hidden disability. This may be from embarrassment, or because the disability has not been fully explained to them. There might also be some jealousy as the child with special needs is often seen to take up too much of a parent's time and interest. So, it is important if one child in the family has ADHD, and seems to the other children to be getting away with murder, to explain the situation to them. One parent told me: 'I explained to my younger son that it was as if his brother had no brakes to put on, and therefore his behaviour went overboard at times.' This will help to explain to one child why there will be a swift punishment for bad behaviour for him while he sees a brother or sister apparently getting away with it.

We hear from the children themselves in chapter 17, but I do know that even very young children begin to get anxious about why they cannot fulfil a task which is impossible for them to fathom out, but which seems so easy to everyone else. This may be exactly the same question the parents are asking themselves. Should the fact that he has a disability, and will on occasion find himself disadvantaged, be conveyed to the child sooner rather than later?

Barry told me that he wished someone had talked to him. All he knew was that he was never sure which hand to use for anything. 'It seemed to me pot-luck whether I used my right or left hand. This means that I was always awkward about playing table tennis, things like that. I just put it down to my stupidity and stopped doing anything where I might get shown up. I missed out on a lot. I never talked to anyone about it.'

Adults who struggled throughout their childhood can recall times when it seemed to them that nobody noticed they had problems. Those who had had difficulties in learning to read remembered how the content meant nothing when they had glossed over words or even whole passages which were incomprehensible to them. The end result was that they were left feeling stupid when they couldn't then answer questions in class. Imagine this happening day in and day out. Many of them recall how in time they began to believe what the other kids called them: 'thick' and 'silly'. Descriptions which hurt just as much as the teachers' delineation of them as 'careless' and 'inattentive' and 'distracted'. Once again all this combined to make the child accept these labels with tremendous loss of self-esteem.

As children grow up and are expected to look after themselves, a hidden disability becomes more obvious. As Steve said: 'I felt physically sick with shock when I finally let myself acknowledge that my 4-year-old never, ever looked me in the eye.' As I said earlier, when a child is very small it is possible to convince yourself that nothing is wrong, and that your child is just a little late in reaching some of the milestones. Remember, that may well be true, and most families have in their folklore a story of an uncle or grandparent who didn't say a word until he was three years old.

We know that some children are late walkers, but it begins to send a chill into any mother's heart when other difficulties start to show: tying shoelaces, using cutlery, doing puzzles, riding a bike – the things which many children delight in mastering – become insurmountable obstacles. Indeed the first thought that 'something is up' may come when a younger child overtakes with ease an older sibling still struggling to dress himself. Peter said he was shocked into thinking about his eldest child when Brian, the 'baby' of the family, asked why Will didn't ever dress himself. Until then, the routine dressing of the children had continued, but when the youngest wanted to do it himself it drew attention to the fact that 6-year-old Will had never tried. Brian began to look for an answer.

'What have I told him? Nothing, he doesn't have the wherewithal to know he is different, and he never asks questions,' said Pamela. However, there are children who do ask, 'What's wrong with me?' This is the perfect opportunity to grasp the nettle and to have a heart-to-heart, so the important thing is to be prepared. If you are not, then the temptation will be to gloss over the cause, and the moment may be lost for ever. If you can encourage your child to talk about his or her worries and what has caused them it may be the time to talk more about strategies which will help. If you can engage your child's attention in understanding more about areas of difficulty, then together you will be able to forge a helpful alliance. It is the child who does *not* ask questions who shows more cause for concern.

Perhaps in our busy grown-up world we neglect the less obvious problems which some of our children have. 'Left-handed? Oh, does that just mean buying a special pair of left-handed scissors?' In fact, it means a great deal more as any left-hander will tell you as playing card games, sewing and knitting can cause problems. Work can get smudged, and things can get spilt more easily. It may be difficult to work out which side a fork or glass is to be placed, and a simple guide like wearing a ring on one finger as a reminder about which hand to use may help. Thank goodness we have moved from the time when children were 'made' to write with their right hand, often with appalling consequences. Our grandparents can tell us horror stories of children who were forced to conform to the 'proper' way to do things. Make sure your child's teacher is aware that your child is left-handed, and that specialist equipment is available. Also, that your child is shown how to position the paper correctly when working, so that there is room for the arm to move inwards as the hand moves across the paper.

Have we progressed so much in other areas? Our children are tested and assessed every inch of the way. Although this helps to pinpoint many areas of concern, it can also shine a light where it is sometimes not needed. Some parents believe that a diagnosis of ADD or ADHD is often agreed on too speedily, and not always by someone qualified to do so. Rebecca: 'I was so stupid. My little boy was always into everything. I told the health visitor and before I knew where we were it was suggested he be put on medication to calm him down. I didn't know what to do. My husband said it was nonsense.' Rebecca went on to tell me how this decision was one they had to face seven years ago. They did not put him on medication, but decided instead to be tighter with boundaries and to keep him fully occupied. The next years were not easy, but they have not regretted their decision. This is a common dilemma for many parents. How is a parent to judge if they have a mischievous full-of-life little boy, or a child who needs a prescribed drug to quieten him down? Do we as a society want children to be easily manageable and forced to concentrate at the expense of everything else, even if the school work they are given is dull or inappropriate?

The parents of a child with special needs will be reluctant to brag about something he did today for the first time, when they know that other children of his age passed that landmark, maybe, three years earlier. Nevertheless, you have every right to celebrate important milestones for you and your child. Why not? Praise for achievement always goes down well with a child. But beware of going over the top with this. Many adults who talked to me about what it was like to grow up with a 'special need' can remember the humiliation they felt when there was a great fuss made about something which the child was all too aware others had accomplished months or years earlier. So don't over-egg the pudding – the child may feel he is being patronized.

What and when to tell your child
- Make sure *you* have accepted your child's difficulties, before trying to explain to him what they are.
- Be prepared for your child's questions and make sure you listen whenever he asks you anything about his disability.
- Talk to your child in a way appropriate to his age – the information will need updating from time to time.
- Listen to the other children in the family – they will have questions to be answered too.
- Be prepared to let your child take part in consultations and discussions.

Letting the family and others know

When do you tell friends, relatives and loving grandparents that your child has a disability which up until now has not been discussed or revealed? When Joan told her parents that Jackie had been diagnosed as possibly dyslexic, the reply was, 'That's good isn't it? Now somebody can teach her to use her cutlery, I don't like it when she uses her fingers.' Joan was appalled that her parents were unable to appreciate just what it had meant to her to say out loud what had been worrying her and her husband for a long time. However, later she was able to accept that they were in shock at the news, and needed time to absorb the implications of this diagnosis for their beloved granddaughter. Perhaps, too, they had in mind discomforting memories of the times they had corrected Jackie at the dining-room table.

What do you say to a stranger who shouts at you for letting your child use a cabin for the disabled on a ferry? This is what happened to the Walker family. When Mrs Walker was trying to persuade her son to go into the cabin and he was throwing a most dreadful tantrum, a man they had never seen before said, 'He's not disabled. Give him a bloody good hiding.' Do you stop, and try to explain? Do you ignore the comments, even though they are so upsetting? All the parents could do was to contain their son who was reacting to a new situation in a predictable way. They decided to leave educating the world for another day.

Richard: 'Every time I tried to tell my parents about the diagnosis for my son, I just choked up, and couldn't do it. It was easier to tell strangers at the school. When I did tell mum and dad I broke down. It was the first time I had cried since I was told my boy is autistic.'

'Don't tell "the world" until you are ready to do so,' said Rachel. 'I told my family and they just said, "Oh dear," and went on with their meal. That hurt. Neither my brother nor my sister have ever talked to me about what it must mean for us all.'

The truth is that people often don't know what to say when they hear the news, and fear of making things worse, or of their own embarrassment, may mean that your announcement is met with silence. Try not to be too hurt by this, and give your friends and family time to adjust to the news.

Helen is a very close friend of a family where the little boy is dyspraxic. She contacted me to ask if I could tell her where to find more information about this condition. Helen was distressed because she could see her friend was worried about her 4-year-old, but she never discussed that he might have a disability. 'We talked about everything under the sun – but never about the way Bob was having co-ordination difficulties.' Helen told me what a relief it was when her friend told her that they had had Bob assessed, and although he didn't fit all the 'criteria' for dyspraxia he certainly walked awkwardly and couldn't skip or hop. Once it was out in the open, Helen felt she could offer her friend some support, and by talking candidly show the family that there was no need to keep it a secret; dyspraxia wasn't a word to hide. Helen said she was interested and would help Bob in any way she could. 'Until we spoke about whether Bob is dyspraxic or not, I felt my friend was slipping away from me.'

What can you do if you are concerned about a child whom you believe needs help and whom the parents do not seem to be concerned about. This can be dangerous ground. The parents may well have some idea that something is not right, and yet not be ready to talk to anyone about the situation. Also, they may feel that it is a private matter and not up for discussion. But, as we have seen earlier, Carrie was shocked when her mother-in-law asked if she was worried about Jennie's daydreaming. We often prevent ourselves seeing something right in front of our eyes if on an unconscious level we are afraid to face up to a situation. So, tread carefully, because you may be moving into an area which is painful and fraught. Beware, too, of sounding critical and using a 'something must be done' approach, even if this has been brought about by your concern and anxiety.

Graham, the father of a child who has Asperger syndrome, contacted me with this bleak comment: 'You will never change people's ignorance however much you talk. They don't want to know about "hidden disabilities". I have told and told the school, and still the teacher complains *every* day that Tom won't concentrate. Tom knows more about Asperger's than his teacher ever will.'

> **Letting the family and friends know**
> - Remember, it is entirely up to you to decide who and when to tell.
> - Make sure you are ready for it when you break the news.
> - People will react in different ways – be prepared for this.
> - Not everyone will understand just what the disability entails, so steel yourself for ill-considered reactions which are wrong and hurtful.

Grandparents' support

If you are reading this book and you are a grandparent – or any other relation – of a child with a special need, you will know that your whole family will have been affected in one way or another. You will also know that the child's parents need all the support they can get. Be prepared for questions such as, 'Do you think there is something wrong with my baby?' and make sure you do not just come up with reassurance. Most young parents fuss and fret, and usually it is over nothing at all, but give a mother or father time to talk about what is worrying them. Reassuring a mother that there is nothing to be anxious about simply because you want to protect her isn't useful. Nor should you dismiss her worries out of hand as she may have noticed something which is not obvious to you yet. If you are asked for advice, and you think there is something to be concerned about – say so. If you are not sure how you can be of use, *ask* if there are any ways you can help

Parents need special support during those early days of 'not knowing' and, as I have already explained, this period can go on for some considerable time. Prepare yourself for a long haul. As Molly said to me: 'Having a grandchild with a hidden disability isn't something that is a one-off thing. The pain and worry go on and on and on.' Ellen: 'My grandson is "borderline" ADHD. We have seen the heartaches that surround this child. He is very bright, yet gets low grades because he cannot sit still to do his work. I believe that positive reinforcement works better than punishment. You have to be sure to channel all that energy in the right direction.'

If you don't understand the nature of the disability your grand-child or nephew or niece may have, make it your business to find out. Be prepared to learn. You may have taken on board that he is 'autistic' or 'ADHD', but do you know what that means? Do you know how to help a child with an emotional outburst? It is often the way the symptoms manifest themselves which is hard to deal with: a child who is dyspraxic is likely to have problems with feeding himself, so brace yourself for the mess at mealtimes if this is something you find hard to watch. If you are concerned about a child who may have ME you will need to cope with knowing that there is no cure and all you can do is support the child in the way that feels best.

If you are the parent, try to bring the grandparents on board. You have probably already found that they can be an inestimable source of support. However, the way you look at your child's special needs, and even the name you give to the symptoms, can cause some tensions between the different generations, so it is as well to be prepared for this. Don't assume that they know what 'developmental delay' or 'Asperger syndrome' means. Explain it to them, and make sure they really do know what can and cannot be expected of your child.

Make sure your parents and in-laws know the difference between SEN (special educational needs) and ESN, the old abbreviation with which they may be familiar which stood for 'educationally sub-normal'; this confusion has distressed many grandparents.

Beryl had no idea that there was any history of autism in her husband's family, yet when listening to her mother-in-law's stories she began to realize that there had indeed been several close relatives who showed some classic signs of autism. As a result the worries she had about her little boy began to take on another dimension, and she pushed harder for a diagnosis. 'I wish I had known earlier about the family history,' she said. So, listen to all the older genera-tion's stories about the family history!

They may also be caught up in a cycle of disbelief that one of *their* grandchildren may be handicapped in any way, and feel that by denying the severity of the symptoms they can push the truth out of their thoughts. Grandparents love to brag about their grandchildren, and they may dread not being in a position to do this. Above all they may not understand what a disability entails. Children with all manner of 'special needs' were treated very differently years ago – when children with totally different disabilities were often put together out of sight in institutions – so grandparents might not have any idea about what is on offer today.

Take into account that they may not understand that many symptoms can be looked at today in a fresh light, that new advances in understanding are made all the time, and help can be found for a child. Be on the look-out, too, not to be upset by veiled hints that there has been 'nothing like this in our family' which can cast a shadow over extended family parties or gatherings when both sides of a family meet up.

Mrs S contacted me to talk about her grandchildren. She said that she could not believe the fuss her daughter made about her two children. 'First there was a hullabaloo to get them into the "right" playschool.' Then Mrs S was outraged because neither of them was reading and writing as well as her daughter would like. Now there was talk about a 'disability'. Mrs S was convinced that it was her daughter's unrealistic expectations which were putting pressure on the children, and consequently on professionals to come up with a diagnosis. 'It is quite, quite wrong to label these children.' Mrs S had a close friend, also a grandmother, who said that her grandson was a difficult child and hard to control, but to say he had an illness was wrong and she would not go along with it. 'He is a very naughty, unruly boy.'

Grandparents often shake their collective heads in dismay at the way children are brought up today. I often heard such observations as, 'They all do too much', 'Whatever happened to them just playing?' 'Nowadays it has to be off to practise one thing then another, or off to that extra class', 'All these young mothers fuss far too much', 'Whoever said that all children have to be up to the mark in everything?' 'If little Johnny isn't first for everything they just look for an excuse.' In one sense they have a point, as it does seem to me that children today have very little time just to be themselves and to relax and play. Of course, I appreciate the value of computers, and I can see the attraction for such things as playstations as the latest must-have toys, but there is a lot to say for the old-fashioned toy box full of dressing-up clothes which allowed children a certain space and freedom to express themselves creatively away from an adult focus. In this world of split families so many children are moved swiftly at weekends and holidays between parents, but if this is happening to your children make sure they have some free time too. Children who do need extra support can find their whole days filled with therapies of different kinds, so remember that play is an important therapy too.

On the other hand, as a grandmother, I am glad to report that there are many, many grandparents who offer a great deal of support and help to parents of children with severe special needs. Caroline: 'My granddaughter has ME. I'll use an old-fashioned word. She is delicate and needs nursing. I can help.' Lisa told me she has every sympathy for her daughter-in-law who is coping on her own with a son, Liam, diagnosed with ADHD. She said that her son, Liam's father, was an undiagnosed ADHD. She had asked for help with him when he was little and been sent away 'with a flea in her ear'. She also believes that her daughter-in-law is an undiagnosed ADHD. But Lisa was thoughtful when she pondered over whether it helped to pinpoint ADHD in Liam's case: 'Would it not be better just to say that Liam takes after his mum and dad?' (It is generally thought in medical circles that 40 per cent of children with ADD or ADHD have one parent with this condition, although most of the parents I was in contact with did not believe this.)

One woman – Christine – is caring for her little nephew who has a severe attachment disorder. To find some support she has started a website, 'Angels who deserve love' (www.communities.msn.co.uk/Angelswhodeservelove), which has become a haven for many grandparents and other family members parenting a child with special needs. It is a site for people who are having severe problems with a child who is adopted, fostered or placed outside of their family due to unforeseen circumstances. On this site there is plenty of information, and a wonderful feeling of warm supportive friendship – and plenty of laughs too.

Pat Blake was at first at a loss to understand why her grandson was distressed and so obviously unhappy as a baby and toddler. As he grew he became very difficult to manage and was equally averse to love or discipline. 'My daughter was too busy trying to cope with him to look for any help, so I took over the research.' Eventually an osteopath suggested sugar intolerance. 'On a sugar-free diet he was transformed in four days,' said Pat. Following this Pat has become very involved with the HACSG (Hyperactive Children's Support Group), and has written a book on *Additive Free Cooking* available through that organization.

I believe that there can be a very strong bond between the older and younger generations, and grandparents often have the time and the patience to mind their grandchild and help him with different skills. All children thrive on undivided attention and for a child who needs one-to-one care all the time this can be a boon to overstretched parents, so don't ignore this help. Just make sure the grandparents (or indeed babysitters as well) know as much as you do about your child's condition.

One of the pitfalls for a parent of a child with special needs is to feel that you must be 'there' all the time. Don't let this happen. If grandparents can take up some of the slack and give you time off, grab it.

Don't be too worried either if the older generation have some different ways of doing things with kids. Trust me, they will work it out together, and you may be surprised to find that a grandfather can find a way of generating an interest in your child which you had not spotted. A grandmother may discover a hobby or pastime which you had not thought would hold your child's attention. One mother on the brink of collapse from strain and worry did agree reluctantly to let her daughter, who had been diagnosed with severe ADD, go to stay with her grandparents for a week. On Helen's return home she seemed calm and happy and the whole family remarked on the change. Helen had truly had a holiday – a break from the never-ending programme to 'engage' her in activities. Time off, in every sense, had helped this little girl to find some inner peace.

Parents are berated on all sides about 'how to bring up baby', and it seems as if nothing is to be left to chance from the moment of preconception. This can often bring down the wrath of on-lookers and, as we have seen, self-recrimination if anything goes wrong. Once upon a time a young mother had only her own mother or mother-in-law to consult. Now bookshops are packed with books offering advice and dire warnings if this or that is not followed through. In his book *Paranoid Parenting* sociologist Frank Furedi points out that parents are besieged by so much information that they are made to 'feel so insecure and fearful about what they don't understand that virtually anything can be turned into a potential childcare crisis'. The point he makes is that fear for children's safety has come to dominate the parenting landscape, and the children are the losers. It is understandable that a parent of a child who needs extra care should be protected from the rough and tumble of the outside world. But don't overdo it, and as Jenny said to me: 'Oh, these young mothers! A little healthy neglect never hurt anyone.'

If your daughter or daughter-in-law is overburdened by ferrying around a child for assessments and appointments she is likely to find that an extra driver is a godsend, so offer to help her. And if you can suggest a way to give the parents an uninterrupted night's sleep, everyone will benefit. Remember, too, that if there are other children in the family a relation who is able and willing to take them out on treats will be much appreciated. It doesn't have to be an expensive outing – often some respite in a quiet environment will be of great value to them, particularly if they have been feeling neglected by all the attention on the sibling with a special need. If finance is a problem for the young family – and often extra services *do* cost money – are you able to help out at all? If you have access to the Internet have a look at Exceptional Grandparents, a site for grandparents with special needs grandchildren (http://clubs.yahoo.com/clubs/exceptionalgrandparents). And don't forget that fun and enjoyment should come into it as well – that's one of the things that grandparents are for!

An excellent source of help and information is Contact A Family, a UK charity which helps families who care for a child with different disabilities and special needs. Ring the helpline on 0208 808 3555 or email at info@cafamily.org.uk. They may be able to put you in touch with local help and facilities, and maybe other families or support groups. Also, contact Parent Partnership Service (www. parentpartnership.org.uk) who will help with impartial information and support to parents and carers of children with special education needs. The National Parents Partnership Network was established under the aegis of the Council for Disabled Children to support the work of the parent partnership services and is funded by the Department for Education and Skills. Each area has its own source but the NPPN holds the contact list. From Sutton Parent Partnership I heard: 'We always ask new referrals if there are any other significant adults involved in a child's care apart from the parents/carers.' So don't hold back from looking for family support.

Siblings

What about the effect on the brothers and sisters of a child with a hidden disability? Although as time goes on the siblings may learn from parental example that there is a child in the family who needs special care and love, the early days may not be so peaceful. It can be hard for any child to accept that there is a brother or sister who gets extra attention and time from the parents. It can be almost impossible for a sibling to understand this, when that child *seems* to get away with stubborn behaviour and *seems* to be able to flout the family rules for no obvious reason.

Parents talk of their anguish about not being able to give the other children enough time when so much has to go into caring for a child with a severe disability. Indeed, where there are physical attacks from a brother or sister with a disability the other children may find themselves left on their own a great deal, and how are they to understand that this may be for their own safety? Those early days where resentment and jealousy run rife can, alas, set the scene for unkind behaviour in later years.

Consider these comments: 'I could never have a party because of Jeremy.' 'I could never bring a friend home because of the way my brother behaved.' 'The other kids at school used to tease me about the way Benny was at school. I hated Benny for that.' 'I could have understood if he had been in a wheelchair or something, but nobody could understand why she behaved like that. My friends thought she was mad.' 'I was actually terrified of my brother when he threw a wobbler.' These are all comments passed on to me from adults who know what it is like to have a sibling with an invisible special need. Treats that other children take for granted − a meal in a restaurant − may be impossible for a family with a child who will run riot in public.

The problem one mother found was that because she had to care most of the time for a daughter with ME, her other daughter regressed into 'baby' behaviour, even though she is ten years old and very bright. On one level, she believed her daughter, Carol-Ann, did understand and was patient with her sister, yet on another level she resented her mother's preoccupation with her sister's illness. 'We were in danger of becoming a disabled family,' said Evelyn. But there are other children who are very compassionate and will struggle to help a less able sibling. Appreciate this concern when they show it, but make sure they do not take on more than they should at such an early age.

Ensure as best you can that you have time off away from your child with special needs, and in this way make a regular date to spend time alone with each of your other children. *All* children have needs.

It is important that you find ways of talking to your children about what is happening, or not happening, to their sibling. At first, tell them in a non-technical way that they will understand, but as they grow older it is important that they have facts and information about a specific condition. They may want to ask whose fault it is. Behind this question is likely to be the fear that somehow they have caused their sibling's problems. By giving clear answers not only will this help them to understand, they will also be properly informed if they are asked by their friends what is happening. Make sure that their teachers know that there are extra pressures at home. Encourage them to talk about their feelings, and listen to their questions. You may have to explain this is a condition which will not go away, and that there are ways for everyone to help. Older siblings may begin to worry about whether they are going to have to look after their brother or sister in the future if their parents die. When trying to answer this question it may be the first time you have let yourself think about the future in this way.

At the very least, by talking about a brother or sister's difficulty you will be signalling that it is nothing to be ashamed of and, as a family, this is something you are all aware of and are all pulling together over.

Dealing with other family members
- Make sure you are ready to talk about your child's disability with the family.
- Be prepared to be met with denial, depression, anger or indifference.
- Prepare yourself with any facts or information you want to share with the other children.
- By talking openly about the condition you will show them that it is not a taboo subject.
- Let them know they can come and ask you questions any time about their brother's or sister's condition.
- Make sure you give regular undivided one-to-one attention to each of your children.
- Don't become so consumed with anxiety about your child that you forget to have playtime too.

Part Two

The Most Common Disorders

5

ADHD (attention deficit hyperactivity disorder)

The mind that has no fixed aim loses itself, for, as they say, to be everywhere is to be nowhere.

(Montaigne, *Essays*)

No simple solution

In this part of the book I devote a chapter to each of the most common hidden disabilities which parents talked to me about. Not only are there more 'invisible' disabilities than I can list, but, as we have seen, all hidden handicaps have differing degrees of severity. Also, from my discussions with parents and carers it has become very clear that the real predicament for many families is that one disability often merges into another.

Parents whose child is put under the 'autistic' umbrella often find that life becomes even *more* perplexing, as there are so many sub-groups. So the diagnosis which they hoped would make things clearer, makes the situation more complicated.

The symptoms

Like so many disabilities, ADHD is characterized by a number of symptoms; and there is a fine line between these and many of the symptoms of ADD, ADHD and the whole autism spectrum disorder. Moreover, a word of warning to start with; the symptoms which point to a diagnosis of ADHD encompass some behavioural indicators which are likely to show themselves in *most* children at one time or another. So, proceed with extreme caution! And note, for instance, that the child with ADHD will sometimes have many of the same difficulties as the child with ADD; the difference is that the child with ADHD is hyperactive.

Some people regard a diagnosis of ADHD as a convenient label for children who are anti-social or just behave badly for one reason or another. But, ADHD is becoming accepted as a genuine disability needing treatment and understanding. This has gone a long way to removing the stigma from parents who up until now have had to battle not only with their child, but with the outside world too; parents who are prepared to stand up and be counted, and some are very vocal in demanding help and treatment for their children.

Hyperactivity can manifest itself in many different ways. First, we need to be clear what hyperactivity can mean. In boys, the most common form is physical hyperactivity, and this can become a general label for different problems ranging from an overall inability to sit still, always being on the move, having a short attention span together with poor short-term memory, plus real difficulties in being able to concentrate long enough to think problems through. Girls are more likely to show a trait of verbal hyperactivity. This divergence is sometimes given as one of the reasons why more boys than girls are diagnosed with ADHD – it is five to seven times more common in boys. Obstreperous and boisterous behaviour draws attention to this disorder, and consequently the cry goes up: 'Something must be done.'

I have been told that having this condition is like a whirlwind in your mind, everything blows around and nothing stays in one place. Being a child, or adult, with ADHD is often compared to trying to watch television as someone changes the channel every few seconds. You have flashes of what is going on, but can't construct the whole picture. People with ADHD tend to dismiss the rules and structures which most people catch onto more readily, and this can leave them feeling totally out of synch much of the time. It is no wonder that frustration grows rapidly and adds to the difficulty of coping with this disorder. It is not directly related to intelligence, so it is important to keep in mind that ADHD occurs in people with IQs on every level.

As I said, any child may well exhibit for a while some of the following signs when he is anxious or distressed. Please do keep this in mind and don't jump to conclusions too quickly. Here is a checklist of the most common characteristics of ADHD:

When a child . . .
- is easily frustrated and distracted
- is disorganized
- has difficulty in remaining seated
- is easily excitable
- talks excessively
- constantly interrupts
- loses things
- engages in dangerous activities without appreciating the consequences
- cannot wait for turns
- is reluctant to share
- has difficulty in planning
- shifts from one activity to another
- is restless
- is fidgety
- has very restless sleep patterns
- is always on the go
- rushes about
- blurts out answers in class
- can't sit still in class or at table
- is inclined to squirm

- cannot play quietly
- has difficulty completing tasks or following instructions
- exhibits lack of persistence
- is inclined to be hyperfocused with limited attention.

This checklist merely provides guidelines, because aren't *all* children 'inclined to squirm', have 'selective attention', and refuse to 'play quietly'? Yes, we all know they do! But, at the other end of the scale depending on their potency and frequency, I have found these signs often do not carry the weight and seriousness they should. If many of these characteristics come together in one child, then caring for that child means total turmoil for the family. Take, at random, some of the symptoms listed. What do they mean in practice?

Can't sit still at table. This is not the fidgety child we all know. It is not the child who gets bored and wants to get down and be off playing. This symptom means that there is not one family meal taken in peace, ever. Banging cutlery, kicking chair legs and brothers and sisters, throwing food, making a noise are just some of the daily pressures which have to be lived with. Sally told me that if she removes Jack from the table for time-out, he will kick the door, wall or anything he can. This has resulted in her eating with Jack, while her husband has his meals separately with their daughters. 'It is splitting up our family,' said Sally. Melinda said that her son taps all the time. He taps on the table, on the plate, on his chair, on the wall as he passes by, and she said that meals taken as a family are quite out of the question, let alone eating in a restaurant or with friends.

Cannot play quietly. This means that a child needs to be constantly entertained or stimulated, and demands one-to-one attention at *all* times. Molly: 'From the moment Alan wakes up it is go, go, go.' Children with this overpowering energy may carry out extraordinary physical tasks. 'He will run up and down the stairs one hundred times without stopping, shouting all the time at the top of his voice,' said Rob.

Cannot follow instructions. Most children are willing to dress themselves most of the time. To put on their own clothes, even if back to front, is seen as a mark of growing up. But, if *every* day your child baulks at putting on underwear, socks and other items of clothing then gentle persuasion and cajoling eventually runs out. There isn't a parent under the stars who has not become exasperated by a child's procrastination, but this is more than that. It is your child never ever doing what he is told. It is never compromising on his part and seeing that you have a point.

Reluctant to share. All children go through a period in their maturational process during which they find sharing toys, or people, difficult. Most people can be tolerant when this applies to a toddler, but when a child is older then the sparks fly. A child with ADHD may show signs of an inability to understand why he or she should share, and if there are other children in the family this can be a constant source of aggravation. Older children may understand that this is a problem and learn to skirt around it. But not a younger child, who will need your protection. Sally told me that every time her little girl played with a toy Jack took it away. Tired of always trying to explain, tired of shouting, Sally found she was putting her daughter in her buggy in a separate room for longer and longer periods. 'I saw she was in danger of becoming an invisible child, but Jack is so attention-seeking that all my energies went on him.' If another child put up any resistance then Jack would lash out, and this was the final nail in the coffin with other mothers; all invitations to play with other kids dried up.

Very restless sleep patterns. This does not mean the occasional bad, disturbed night, familiar to all parents of a baby or young child. It means living with a child who may seem to need only five hours sleep a night, every night. Lisa told me that her grandson Liam has slept badly since he was one day old. He cried constantly as a baby if put down, and was three years old before he could sleep for a few hours at a stretch. Even now he only sleeps about five, or maybe six, hours a night. She often gets a phone call from her daughter-in-law at ten or eleven o'clock at night, or very early in the morning, for someone to go and help her. It is always chaos when he wakes – which can be at five in the morning – until his medication kicks in. This lack of peaceful sleep was one of the things parents reported as a major problem.

Children with ADHD find it most difficult to focus their attention for any length of time and almost impossible to regulate their behaviour, and knowing and accepting this does not make it any easier to cope with. In class, the behaviour of a child with ADHD can become a torture for the teacher, the other children and in many cases for the child himself. At home there may never be a quiet moment and the child's level of activity can wear out the most loving and attentive families. Too many parents are at the end of their tether. Molly summed it all up in four words: 'I cannot go on!'

Parents speak

'Help. Help. Please find me some help,' said Elsie. A national newspaper had run an article on 'A terrifying illness – ADHD'. Parents were invited to contact the newspaper if they had 'a problem child with no hope of help'. When Elsie finally spoke to the journalist she was told that there had been 'too many calls' and no more were being taken. Elsie was devastated, because she had hoped that help would be at hand. She contacted me and told me a most harrowing tale. Her 9-year-old boy had shown signs of great activity from the age of three and was soon excluded from nursery school for beating up other children. 'The school kicked him out too,' she went on. 'And, at home he runs riot.' I asked what this really meant. The catalogue of events she reported was frightening. He had attacked their dog with a pitchfork and the animal had to be put down, he killed their guinea pig, threw the kitten down the stairs, and regularly beats up his little brother – the 5-year-old Timmy is 'covered in bruises'.

Sally told me that her son Jack has a very high IQ, which she believes makes his condition of ADHD even more difficult for him.

She also considers that because she knows he is bright it is harder for her, with the inevitable daily battles about getting up, getting dressed, into the car, out of the car . . . the list is endless. Anthea, whose son is also bright, has a similar problem: the school will not agree to him being statemented. This means there is no additional help for him, although the school constantly complains about his disruption in class. John has been diagnosed as having ADHD by a psychiatrist, but the diagnosis has not brought the family much support. Anthea said any parent of a child with ADHD must be prepared to 'fight, fight and fight'. She went on to say: 'I am up and down to the school all the time. I had no idea at the beginning what a long drawn out battle it would be. When I first went to my GP five years ago for help, he didn't even know what ADHD was and I had to get some leaflets from America for him to read! He was still very sceptical though. So, tell anyone to get their child evaluated by appropriate people, not the school or a GP. It has to be a psychiatrist.'

Again, it is imperative that parents should understand that most children will display some of the symptoms associated with ADHD, usually to a lesser degree. It is only when they are *so pervasive and disruptive* that the name ADHD should be given, and then only by someone qualified to do so. The time to be concerned is when your child's behaviour is *significantly* different from his peers, and when it shows in *more than one setting*. Not, for instance, just at school. And, only when this behaviour has manifested itself for *at least six months*.

'Six months?' cried Sally. 'I have been trying to get help since Jack was two. It has been two and a half years of hell. I have screamed for help. When I was told he was on yet another six-months waiting list to be seen for another assessment I cried. I was told it was because there were children with greater needs. I rang up and shouted at them, "Do you want me to bring him into the casualty department with two broken arms, because that is what will happen. There is a mother and child in crisis here." I got an appointment within a week, but it is terrible that it had to come to that.'

Another mother who contacted me to talk about her son and ADHD said that she knew from the time Frank was a small boy that he had some kind of disability. This little boy walked at ten months, and by just over a year was climbing trees with no regard for any danger. However, she fought against the diagnosis of ADHD because she felt it had been too widely used and often masked bad parenting and disobedient children.

Stella told me that one of the difficulties of living with a child with ADHD is that you have to be very clear all the time about what you are saying. 'Hold on for five minutes' must mean just that, not ten or fifteen minutes. 'I may take you to the shops later' means to the child that you will take him to the shops. 'There is no leeway,' she said, 'and that can be very exhausting.'

From Stella I heard that living with a child with the disorder can be very, very trying. The up-side is that Frank is fun to live with, and because he has such a high energy level, he can be a bit of a clown. 'His friends see him as Jack the lad.' But, I soon understood from what Stella said that it can be very draining to live with a family member who is clowning around one moment, but in a terrible rage the next. 'Rude', 'disruptive' and 'troublesome' were adjectives used to describe him. 'But,' said Stella, 'we have never, ever given up on him.'

Stella believes that her son never knew what it meant to concentrate. On the rare occasions he became absorbed in a book, for instance, she made it her business to comment on how *that* was concentrating. 'We had to teach him.'

Like many other parents Stella felt that her other, older son has missed out on a lot. Frank took up all their time and energy, and, just to keep the peace, what Frank wanted Frank often got. Eventually when Frank was thirteen a psychologist formally diagnosed ADHD, and by that time Stella and Bill accepted it, in the hope that there would be extra help for him. This did not happen. He was not statemented, and received no extra help at school. Fortunately, Frank was popular with the other children, being an excellent sportsman helped a great deal.

Stella was one of the first parents to talk to me about Ritalin. She is sure that taking this drug made Frank calmer and better able to cope with his school work. But he did not like 'the way it made me feel' – this is a very common complaint from children – so he stopped taking it. As Stella and Bill have concluded that ADHD is untreatable, they decided that Frank must make his own decision about his medication, and he must find his own way of living with this condition. To the surprise of the school, Frank has passed his A-level exams, but cannot settle to make applications for college or further education. He is too restless to plan his future. Stella and Bill are now standing back, because having supported him for seventeen years, they feel he must make the next decisions for himself. 'Now it is time for him to take responsibility for his life,' said Bill.

I asked about support over the years from friends and family. Stella sighed and said Frank had been 'too much' for the wider family, and as for friends, 'They just used to laugh at the impossible things Frank said and did.' Stella and Bill both agreed that without the strong support of each other, they would never have coped over the years.

Wendy urged me to caution parents about being too hasty. Her son ran into trouble at school, and although she found no problems with him at home she was under great pressure from the school for him to see a psychiatrist. Wendy said that she dug her heels in and took him to see a therapist instead. What emerged was that there were problems at school, but ones which could be ironed out without medication; and counselling, plus family therapy, put her son back on course. 'We listened to him, and gave him much more time. And he did have a grievance at school which nobody knew about.' Wendy and her husband both agreed they were fortunate in having the chance to tap into other resources because without counselling they may well have gone down the medication route.

I heard from Barry, whose son was also always 'on the go', that a child who has the symptoms which often lead to a diagnosis of ADHD can sometimes be a delight to be with. A high energy level can at times be a plus, and can motivate others to get involved with a project. The difficulty arises when the interest fades and the child is off on another scheme before one task is complete. 'I can't count the innumerable times he has started a school newspaper, wanted to put on a play or organize a bring-and-buy. And then moved on to another interest. Luckily, he can charm his friends into doing the work.'

As with most 'invisible' disabilities there is often disagreement about whether ADHD is a handicap or not. Harold would not believe that his son should be treated in any way for his behaviour. He said that as a boy he himself had been hyperactive and that it had never troubled him, and for that reason he blocked any attempt by the school to discuss ways that Kenny might be helped. When Kenny was in trouble for causing uproar at school, Harold told them to get on with disciplining him, since that was the way he himself had been handled. 'Boys will be boys,' he said. 'Why do we all want children to be the same? They are not.'

At first Elsie got some help in London, but a move to another part of the country meant that there was no help on offer. In fact, she had to start from square one, and she found the professionals were looking to her to explain what ADHD was! She told me that the chaos brought about by Robert is causing the total break-up of the family. 'Last night I woke to find Robert standing by my bed and pissing all over me. That's the sort of thing he does all the time.' Her real worry is that he threatens to kill his brother, or himself, and often dashes into the road in the face of oncoming traffic. 'I must have help,' said Elsie. 'A social worker is coming to see me, but she rang me yesterday and she asked if he is autistic. She didn't seem to know anything about ADHD. What am I going to do?' Elsie had searched for assistance locally and she did find a group, but they seemed primarily interested in getting their children prescribed Ritalin 'because then the child is seen as disabled and you are entitled to claim some money'.

Disruptive behaviour and discipline

My telephone rang again immediately after my conversation with Elsie. Barbara had spoken to me before and she wanted to give me an update on her son. He had begun school two months previously and after initial chaos had, to some extent, settled down. She believed the school, from day one, made sure he was kept busy. However, at home he was markedly worse, and at weekends they had to go out in the car from nine in the morning until bedtime. It was the only way they could contain him. At home, his two younger sisters were on the receiving end of his bullying and attacks. Barbara, too, wanted to talk about her boy's reaction to Ritalin.

So, how can a parent help their child? Once a parent finds that ordinary parenting strategies have no impact upon their child, morale suffers and they are totally demoralized. When parents are in step with their child, then parenting should be a delight and an okay job. When this does not happen and parents feel ignored or powerless it is hard to change to different strategies. However, above all you must be consistent in the rules you make, and it is important that both parents agree on the approach that is being taken. It is not surprising that one of the most difficult areas for parents of a child with special needs is that of discipline. Can there be too much? Or too little?

If you have been cowed over the years by your child's tantrums, it is hard to begin to draw the line and to deal with the anticipated explosion when you tell your child to do something. Too many of the parents I was in contact with had thrown in the sponge where discipline was concerned, and who could blame them? To be faced eyeball to eyeball with a child with severe signs of ADHD or PDA can be a frightening experience. Parents often felt that the battle was lost, and, as one father told me, 'If I laid a finger on Ralph I would really have laid into him and broken every bone in his body.' However, if every domestic issue becomes a screaming battle where nobody wins, the family is in a state of war twenty-four hours a day.

Children with ADHD appear to be so demanding that they can easily drain any adult's energy, so that a situation can quickly develop where the more the child wants from a parent, the less the parent feels inclined to give. Flora said that Thomas demands constant one-to-one attention from the moment he wakes. With two other children and a home to run Flora is often unable to 'give' any more, and so to protect herself and her other children, she cuts herself off from her son. This, of course, means that he makes more and more demands. This spiral of attention-seeking has meant that Flora has collapsed under the strain and has twice been admitted to a psychiatric hospital with severe depression. 'He is a lovely boy really and if I had all the time in the world to give him, I think he would be all right.' As a mother on her own she can see the dreadful impact all this is having on her other children.

So, how best to help your hyperactive child? For each desperate parent who spoke with me, there were others fired with enthusiasm about the way they were able to help their child. They range from parents prepared to accept that they have a *very* overactive child who needs and demands constant one-to-one attention, to those who vow that medicating a child is the only – and the best – way of helping. Others say a strict diet brought about improvement, and yet others that only a tight set of boundaries will contain a child with the symptoms of ADHD, while unfortunately there are those who remain lost in the midst of trying different strategies and finding they do not work for their child.

The one thing all of them would agree on, though, is that there is insufficient help for parents who are desperate to find the *right*, and best, way of helping their child.

The use of medication

There is widespread disagreement about the use of medication for children. And when it comes to ADHD one is really talking exclusively about Ritalin. It has now been prescribed for over forty years and is the most common medication parents told me about, although some mentioned Dexedrine, Concerta Cylert and Adderall, and a number of children were even prescribed a cocktail of drugs. One newspaper report claimed that one-third of schoolboys in America are taking Ritalin, another asserted that 3.8 million schoolchildren have been prescribed regular medication. In the UK, where it is estimated that 4 per cent of children in England and Wales have severe hyperactivity, drugs have been licensed for its treatment where non-drug measures alone have proved insufficient. The first choice is for behavioural and educational approaches, and stimulant drugs are only prescribed when the disorder is severe, or for children who cannot tolerate other treatment. The policy stated by most health authorities is that drug treatment is only given when a child has failed to respond to other forms of therapy or when the condition is very severe and the child is disabled. However, from the parents I interviewed, it was evident that non-drug measures are *not* always the first treatment of choice by professionals. Many parents I met were desperate for alternative or additional help.

ADHD is more frequently diagnosed in the US than in the UK or Europe, and medication is used more rapidly there than in other countries, although the different approaches to the various disorders in many countries makes it impossible to form a completely coherent picture. I understood that in Japan the number of children with ADD/ADHD is negligible, but whether this was because of diagnosis or diet was not clear to me. I later found that in Japan there is aid only for children recognized as having autism/Asperger syndrome provided they have 'mental retardation' as well. For help to be offered the IQ must be below 50. This leaves a vast number of children – and their parents – in limbo. Today, in all parts of the world, mostly because parents have searched the Internet for help, there is growing awareness about other conditions and a greater demand for help for children.

Ritalin is a stimulant since it increases or stimulates overall brain activity. Those in favour of Ritalin believe that this drug helps children to control their impulses and to enhance their concentration and short-term memory. By using it, children are more capable of calming down, and can communicate more easily with their peers. But even the most fervent advocate of stimulant medication will agree that it does not suit every child for whom it is prescribed.

Parents have become concerned when their child shows signs of insomnia – an acknowledged side effect – and another drug has been added to combat this. Some have also told me that it was not 'calming' they noticed but depression, with the consequence that an antidepressant was added to the cocktail of drugs prescribed for the child.

Any newspaper or magazine article about Ritalin is usually prefaced by describing it as 'the controversial drug Ritalin', but for many parents there is no quarrel and they welcome the difference Ritalin has made to their child's behaviour and life.

'Bryan has had a good response to medication. We don't give it to him consistently, but he does ask for it if he is having a particularly hard day. It calms him down right away and helps him deal socially better. I think it is because he can slow down his mind and think things through first.'

Many other parents also said that their child does not need medication all the time, and as the medication does not therefore build up in their system, there are no withdrawal signs. 'Sometimes Ben gets med. twice a day . . . sometimes it is a month or more before he gets a single one. I base it on what he needs, what I'm observing, and what he tells me. In that order.'

I heard from families who were on their knees before medication was prescribed. One mother said that one tablet in the morning brought almost instant calm, and a slow-release dose at the same time meant that the school day could be got through. 'Before the slow-release Ritalin was available there was chaos from lunchtime onwards at school.' But, as there was no nurse on the premises Alec had to remember to take the tablet. As a child, he would 'forget' or think he didn't need it, with disastrous consequences. The school was uncooperative in helping with medication, but, said Vikki, they were quick enough to be on the telephone to tell me he had just walked out of class or caused a fight.

'Ritalin. Are you joking? Five years ago I would have had a word or two to say about any parent who gave their child a drug day in and day out. Today I see it quite differently, and if it were not for Ritalin I would have either killed myself or my son by now. Seriously.'

Lisa told me that she thinks slow-release Ritalin is 'brill'. Liam no longer gets the high in the middle of the day he used to get on ordinary Ritalin, and he doesn't have to take medication at school which saves him embarrassment and relieves him from having to remember to take it. There is a great deal of control over how and where this drug can be prescribed. 'Liam's 'script is locked in a safe until we can pick it up.' This is because slow-release Ritalin is not yet licensed in the UK and great caution is taken over prescribing it. There are horror stories going around about children selling their medication to other kids at school.

Annie, too, said that after four years of desperately seeking help for her son she had reluctantly decided to give Ritalin a try. Every other avenue had been explored and she felt she was in danger of physically harming her boy in an effort to contain him and to get him to slow down. She told me that unless you live with a child with ADHD and the chaos he causes – never letting the family have a meal in peace, hitting out at the other children *all* the time – you have no right to criticize a parent who goes for medication in an effort to calm things down. 'It's either that or I shall harm him, or myself.'

Timmy, now fifteen years old, told me that 'Ritalin's okay'. He only takes it during school term time 'because it slows me down so that I can think', but he does not see the need for it at weekends or holidays. Do his friends know he takes medication? 'If they ask, I tell them.'

Timmy went on to say that as a small boy he can remember having so much energy he thought he would burst and he had to rush around all the time. He didn't know he had a problem, but he was aware that he had more energy than other children.

Bob, too, at fourteen years old, said that he felt better when on Ritalin, of which he takes three doses each day. He said that the school are very discreet about handing out his medication at lunch-time, and on a school trip it was all organized for him. Bob said that at weekends he sometimes forgets and then both he and his family soon know about it as he begins to rock and tap and generally be disruptive. He remembered that when he first started taking Ritalin he had no appetite and lost weight, but his mum found that if he ate at the same time as taking the tablet the food went down. If they waited for the Ritalin to take effect he was not hungry.

Pros and cons of Ritalin

For every parent who was grateful for the change they saw once their child was on medication, there was another parent who fiercely opposed any drug treatment. 'We teach our kids to say NO to drugs, and then pump them full of medication. That cannot be right,' said Kevin.

'Ritalin does not help, and while parents use this as a band-aid treatment, the real issues are not being discussed.' Ron was vehement in his campaign against medication for children with ADHD. 'Can't parents see that it may remove certain symptoms of behaviour but it does not address the underlying problem. How can any parent give their child a drug which is classified by the American Drug Enforcement Agency as a substance which has the same pharmacological effects as cocaine?' 'The side effects that kids have need watching. Poor appetite is par for the course.' 'Putting my boy onto a drug was my last hope. It didn't help, in fact it speeded up everything, except what was needed. It has speeded up his emotions, and he can't control them – he fusses like a 2-year-old over something trivial, and then cries uncontrollably for an hour.'

Elsie said that in desperation she agreed that her son should have Ritalin. 'Oh my God, it made things worse. First of all his brothers teased him about taking it so there was a terrible fuss to make him have it. Sometimes I would hide it in his food. But he always said it made him feel sick, and I couldn't see any improvement in his behaviour. Sometimes he was sick. So I stopped it.'

Barbara used Ritalin as a 'last resource' for her son and was devastated when it did not work in the way she had been led to believe it would. He seemed a little calmer after a dose, but as it wore off he was much more out of control than before. Also, he cried a lot, had tremendous pressure of speech – would talk non-stop for up to three hours at a time – and became very clingy. Both these mothers were distraught to find that 'the last resort' had not lived up to expectations. They both felt there was nowhere else to turn.

A legal battle rages in the US between a school and some parents who want to take their child off the medication because of the drug's side effects, which include sleeplessness and loss of appetite. The school called in the child protection services alleging child abuse when the parents said they wanted their child taken off the drug. They are being forced into court to clear their name. There are other lawsuits in process charging that drug companies have 'deliberately, intentionally, and negligently promoted the diagnosis of ADD/ADHD and sales of Ritalin through its promotional literature and through its training of sales representatives'. The suit also charges that the manufacturer of Ritalin financially supports some organizations which promote and support the ever-increasing implementation of the ADD/ADHD diagnosis as well as directly increasing Ritalin sales.

Patsy, with two very hyperactive boys, said that she tried everything under the sun – except drugs. She went against the advice of the school, her doctors and her family; she refused to accept that a regular use of any drug is the right way to help a child. Nor was she the only parent I heard from who voiced their apprehension about this 'quick fix'. They felt that although a child on Ritalin may fit in more with the family and community, it did not always mean that this was in the best interest of the child. It is a boon for many desperate end-of-their-tether families just because it is 'fast acting'.

Jane told me that her brother was exceedingly hyperactive, but a later diagnosis moved from ADHD to 'learning difficulties'. In the meantime he was prescribed Ritalin, but he cried whenever he had to take it; he hated the side effects so much.

Doreen told me that her 10-year-old son has been taking Ritalin for five years. 'It has kept our entire family sane,' but it was becoming less effective. The school had reported an inability to concentrate again, and she was fearful that it would mean that an increase in both Ritalin and Luvox (an antidepressant). 'Do we just go on and on increasing the dose?' Yet another parent not able to get advice about what to do for the best.

Bess said that her fear was whether ADHD was a right diagnosis and if so was Ritalin the right medication. Her son did not react well to this medication and it had now been changed. However, although for a couple of hours after taking the new drug he was calmer and quieter, as the effect of the drug wore off 'he was worse than ever. It is as if something has got stored up in him and then had to burst out.' But Bess is a desperate mother too. She says that holidays are a nightmare, 'that things were so bad the last long summer school holiday that I cried every day'. She cannot let him out to play with other kids: 'If I do, then within five minutes he is in a fight. The other kids goad him and he reacts.' I asked what she did with him when he came home from school. 'I lock him in his room,' she said. 'They will hand out a prescription quickly enough, but he needs a lot more help than that. Because he has a high IQ they will not statement him and he has no special help. We are in limbo, can you help us?' Bess needed to talk and talk. I have mentioned what has happened, or rather what has not happened for Richard, but I am sorry to say this story was repeated to me in one way or another over and over again. 'He breaks any toy given to him or to his brothers.' 'He has smashed the telly three times.' 'He terrorizes his brother and sister.' This is what Sally meant when she told me earlier that children with ADHD are more than just 'overexcited'.

'I won't let him have Ritalin, and because I won't let Micky have "a recognized drug for hyperactivity" they have rejected our claim for DLA (Disabled Living Allowance). He does have gamolenic acid and this is actually recommended for hyperactivity by the British Medical Board but not good enough for the DLA office. They don't count diets. Because he does not see a psychiatrist he is not seen as disabled.' This was said by one of the parents who spoke about the efficacy of gamolenic acid.

'No, no, no! I will not let my child be drugged,' a cry from a desperate father. His son's school pointed to ADHD when Alan's behaviour was seen as 'out of order'. But Bill was not convinced that it was anything more than just over-zealous and enthusiastic behaviour. He delved deeply into research on stimulants and he likens the medication prescribed today for ADHD children to the frightening use of Benzedrine years ago for asthma. Bill asked me if I knew that Ritalin carries with it a warning that it 'should not be used in children under six years'. Bill had spoken to many parents of young children who were unaware of this. 'What else are we not being told?' he asked. Meanwhile, he went on looking for different help for his son but realized in the end that it had to come from the family. They found plenty of ways to keep Alan occupied and burn off his surplus energy. Bill: 'Hard work, but worth it.'

'Oh yes, drugs work okay,' said Tim. 'But they produce robotic and zombie-like behaviour in children. No way is my son having any of that. Have you *read* about what the drugs do to the brain? Have you?'

The anti-drug doctor

The dilemma for so many parents is what they should believe of all the comment available to read. A strong body of them have combined their voices to stress the importance of wanting more help with the behavioural and school problems of their children without resorting to drugs. They consider that a mind-altering drug can never be an appropriate approach to helping children.

Dr Breggin, who wrote *Talking Back to Ritalin,* urges parents to 'educate – don't medicate'; he maintains that this should be the motto of all parents and teachers. Dr Breggin is a psychiatrist in the US and he is never afraid to speak out against drugs for children. His concern is about society's double values: at the same time as campaigning to 'Say *no* to drugs' we are prescribing far too many addictive drugs for our children. Breggin believes that the wide availability of prescribed stimulants has led to their increasing illegal use by children and young people. He asks, 'Does a drug become safe simply because it is prescribed by a doctor? Does pushing drugs on children become legitimate simply because it is done by drug manufacturers?'

Breggin holds that, 'It is difficult to distinguish between a child who has an attentional problem and a child who isn't getting enough attention, or between a child who has a discipline problem and a child who isn't getting appropriate discipline.' He thinks that they are one and the same and feels that we, as adults, must make it our job to provide more attention or better discipline rather than to assume the problem lies with the child. This is not to say that he blames the parents, in fact he states quite clearly that he does not: 'I try to help them overcome their feelings of guilt.' Indeed he considers the blame lies with the professionals who are too quick to diagnose ADHD, ADD etc., and for medication to be seen as the 'solution' is quite wrong and leans towards abuse of our children. He feels that the child who is especially sensitive, physically precocious, daring, independent, energetic or creative is at special risk of supposedly having a disorder. Breggin says that anyone who has raised or taught children knows that the most interesting and exciting children are often the most trying. He reminds us of an ancient Greek saying, 'The wildest colts make the best horses.' Whether or not you put your faith in medication, you should take a look at Dr Breggin's passionate anti-drugs views which are available on the Internet on www.breggin.com/ritalin.html.

Medication and managing behaviour

On the other hand, as I have said already, I have had numerous contacts with parents who have told me they could not have gone on a moment longer if their child had not been prescribed medication. 'It helped us to be a family again.' 'School work became possible.' 'I got my son back within a few days of him starting Ritalin.' Sarah told me that when her son was seven years old and prescribed Ritalin, he suddenly put out his hand and held hers for the first time. Some parents reported their children developed facial tics when on slow-release Ritalin, but those on the other side claim the children may have developed them anyway. Just one more point of controversy for a worried parent to fret about.

I don't think anyone believes that medication is a substitute for behavioural management, parental education and support, but help in these areas is woefully under-resourced. It seems to me that the term ADHD in particular is widely and often indiscriminately used. This can lead to parents being told that the only way to help their child is to medicate. I believe it has become an umbrella term and used too speedily, which means that there are many parents totally at sea, looking for help but unsure what they are seeking.

If there has been a *reliable* diagnosis the best way forward for most seems to be a multi-modal treatment approach tailored to the needs of each child. I have been told it is irresponsible even to hint that medication is questionable, and that to hold back on anything which helps a child with this condition is likened to withholding insulin from a child diagnosed with diabetes.

It does seem as if for *some* children medication may be the best and only option. But, as we have seen, ADHD medications do not work for everyone; and statistically 51 per cent of children on Ritalin gradually discontinue it within about four years, for a number of reasons. However, I must also report that it has helped some severely impaired children and enabled them to lead more normal lives. It is the children who cannot tolerate Ritalin, or whose parents do not want to go along the medication route, who are left out in the cold when no other help is offered.

Although the drug Ritalin has been available for treatment of hyperactivity for many years, controversy surrounding its use and wide variation in availability recently brought it to the attention of NICE. (NICE – The National Institute for Clinical Excellence – is an authority set up to give advice on best clinical practice to National Health Service clinicians. It is a key part of the UK Government's plans to ensure quality in the NHS.) The main conclusion was that Ritalin should be used as part of a comprehensive treatment programme for children with a diagnosis of severe ADHD. However, the report also stated that the drug should be discontinued if improvement of symptoms is not observed after appropriate dose adjustments over one month. In addition, it was stated that children on Ritalin therapy should receive regular monitoring, and that the diagnosis should be made on a comprehensive assessment *by a specialist*. This drug is not currently licensed for, among other things, children under the age of six, or for children with marked anxiety, agitation or tensions, epilepsy, Tourette syndrome, or psychotic disorders.

The treatment and care of children with ADHD in the UK is the responsibility of child and adolescent mental health services and a policy statement shows that more money is to be allocated to this under-funded service. Meanwhile the ADHD National Alliance (www.cafamily.org.uk) is concerned that any delay in providing services for the 48,000 school-aged children who have severe ADHD and who are currently undiagnosed and untreated is likely to be very damaging. These stark statistics are contained in the NICE report.

The NICE guidelines suggest a comprehensive treatment programme should involve advice and support to parents and teachers, but need not include specific psychological treatment, such as behavioural therapy. They recommend that while this wider service is desirable, any shortfall in provision should not be used as a reason for delaying the appropriate use of the medicine. This seems to me to be an unfortunate let-out clause for the failure to provide other services needed.

Although the ADHD National Alliance is not a national support group, it promotes and develops new work being carried out across the country by support groups, parents, families and professionals. They work to raise awareness of ADHD and to enable members to share their skills, knowledge and experience. Jim Hedgeland is the co-ordinator on 020 7608 8760.

For and against medication
- Get all the information you can so you can decide whether this is the right course for your child.
- Medication can help *some* children by controlling impulses, improving concentration and short-term memory.
- There are side effects and so medication is not an appropriate treatment for *all* children.
- You need to decide whether it is a 'godsend' or a 'quick fix' for *your* child.

Alternative solutions

Again and again I was told that the general feeling is that many GPs are set in their ways and will not consider trying different solutions for the different disabilities. Edna told me that at first Ritalin helped her son to settle at school, but within a short time the advantages had worn off. He became bad tempered, lost weight and when they returned to their doctor they were told to 'up' the dosage. This didn't seem right to them and they started vitamin supplements. He is now drug free. However, Edna also said that she is not pro- or anti-drugs, and if they work, then that is better than leaving a child untreated. It is just that medication did not help her son.

The consensus of opinion seems to be that medication alone should not be the first or the sole line of help. Some parents have found that both clinical and educational psychologists have been prepared to explore other possibilities. Also, some doctors will work with parents to look for a 'natural' approach which includes nutritional supplements and vitamins and a more holistic or homeopathic course. There are parents who have found that great improvements can be made with a changed diet and correction of any nutritional deficiencies. Artificial colouring, preservatives, flavour enhancers and even some natural chemicals were all given as factors affecting children's behaviour. Some parents swear that diet plays a very large part in managing ADHD and that their children become very restless and irritable when taking certain foods. It seems that there are children who have a very sensitive chemical reaction. Fizzy drinks are often singled out.

Vitamin supplements are another bone of contention. As we heard from Edna, they helped her child, while other parents have spent 'a fortune' on supplements without success.

EFAs (essential fatty acids), on the other hand, are nutrients that are needed for the body, and especially for the brain to function as effectively as possible. A lack of EFAs can also result in dry skin and hair, and brittle nails. These nutrients are found in many foods, especially oily fish. There has been a wealth of research into the relationship between EFAs, zinc and developmental disorders, but many of them have been inconclusive. Much comment has been focused on the possible connection between these supplements and children with ADHD, an area where discussion rages yet again, with the media going on about a 'startling breakthrough in treatment'. But at present there is no scientific evidence to show that it helps. However, I heard from parents who swear that they saw a change in their child's behaviour once they were given regular doses of EFA supplements.

Other parents told me about the HACSG (Hyperactive Children's Support Group) for hyperactive, allergic and learning-disabled children. This organization maintains that attention to diet, by eliminating additives, chemicals and some foods, plus supplementing the diet with important nutrients, can make a considerable improvement. They draw attention to the research at the Institute of Child Health, and other investigations which have found that artificial colours and preservatives came top of the list for causing the problems associated with ADHD.

The database of HACSG shows some basic foods come high on the list of offending items: cow's milk, oranges, wheat and chocolate. One interesting detail I noticed in the HACSG's literature is their statistics show not only that more boys than girls are hyperactive, but that the ratio is 3:1 with a higher percentage of blond blue-eyed boys than the average. HACSG is a charity, now twenty-four years old, and they will give advice about diet/food and chemical intolerance. They promote the Feingold Food Programme, and their handbook, which includes details of the programme, costs £4.00. Visit their website (www.hacsg.org.uk), from which it is possible to download and print out a list of 'E' numbers which you can keep in your pocket. They also have pages of information about different additives to food and drink.

Marie joined HACSG because although she did not believe that diet *caused* ADHD, she did find that her son's condition was aggravated by what he ate. 'There is no doubt he is calmer when I am careful about what he eats,' she said.

Irene said that once she embarked on an elimination diet (foods are restricted and new foods are added gradually to watch for any reaction) the results were astounding. Kevin still did not sleep and was still overactive, but he was calmer, happier and much less destructive. She consulted a dietician to make sure he was receiving a balanced diet. To her later dismay, Kevin was prescribed a high-protein drink, which she soon discovered was made mainly from peanuts which he cannot tolerate! He was also prescribed a zinc supplement which wasn't suitable for him, but she found an alternative, which points to the need for caution on all fronts.

Even if your child responds to a restricted diet there may be problems ahead. Catherine asked if she could meet the school cook, who looked at the list with horror and said that all the meat they cook has additives. Although the school is meant to serve a healthy balanced diet the food is processed. 'Even when they serve a "roast" it is processed and full of "E" numbers.' Catherine said she understood that it is compulsory for schools to provide meals that are suitable for children on special diets – whether for health or religious reasons. 'The cook said she will look into it. So it's packed lunches, which we cannot afford, although he is entitled to a free school meal. And so one more fight ahead, I suppose.'

'I took my child to see a homeopath, but she said there was no magic remedy to help children. In fact she seemed more concerned about me, that I was getting no support with my 5-year-old who had been excluded from school in his first term.' I spoke to this homeopathic doctor; she confirmed that she was seeing a huge rise in the number of children diagnosed with ADHD. 'Was this', she asked me, 'because the diagnosis is being made more readily today?' She felt her hands were tied, and that more resources should be poured into giving support to the despairing parents she sees.

Desperate to find help for her son, Wendy took him to see an osteopath. A friend's child had been helped by having cranial osteopathy treatment and Wendy could see the evidence that the little boy was calmer and happier. However, there was no improvement in her boy's behaviour. 'Another disappointment, another costly try, but we can't afford to leave any stone unturned.'

Other parents believe that professional counselling or

psychotherapy for their child, together with support for themselves, has brought about benefits. A behaviour modification programme – if available – which establishes firm boundaries at home and at school can be very beneficial in supporting a child. This works if there is a strong link between home, school and the service provider. Positive reinforcement through praise helps some children, from which they learn that good behaviour brings rewards. If this is the way forward for your child, it is often hard to persevere if there are no immediate signs of improvement, but do not expect overnight changes. Again, this is where support for the parents is so important, and whatever route they choose, this is always what most families ask for. Grace and Hugh said they could never have succeeded without the back-up of each other, but they did not waver, and believe that now life is at least calm enough for the family to cope again. If you need some professional input seek out a child psychologist or child psychotherapist who has experience working in this area with children.

Another alternative I heard about was from families who had separately reached the conclusion that as there was no help on offer from the outside world, it had to come from inside the home. They devote their days (and often nights) to helping their child through the terrible tantrums and outbursts. They do not take their child to the homes of people who do not understand what is happening, and in this way circumvent 'scenes'. They enlist the help of sympathetic friends and relations who make sure that there is always one-to-one help on hand for their child. Ian told me that there is no doubt they have had six years of hell but, with fingers crossed, they may now be coming out the other side. The times of relative calm were increasing, and they felt that by accepting their child as he is, and by standing by him at all times, the worst might be over for them all. 'Instead of spending all the time on the phone looking for help, I gave what I could to my son. Do tell other parents about us.'

'Everyone has told me that my son has ADHD. I don't really go along with it, but I have tried Ritalin. He hates it and runs away when he sees I have some. But because I was told he should have it I have tried to trick him at times. Oh, the fights we have had. Today, though, out of the blue the doctor said to me, "Perhaps he doesn't have ADHD – let's re-think this medication." I went home and cried my eyes out. Does that mean I have to start all over again?' Tracy, in despair, telephoned me to tell me of this latest in a saga of seeking help for her son.

Worrying reports from the school about 9-year-old Pete, and a suggestion from a teacher about a possible diagnosis of ADHD, had Andrew and Alice searching for help. They believed, quite rightly, that this is not a diagnosis to be made lightly or by somebody not qualified to do so. Both parents lead very busy working lives, both travelling because of work commitments, and taking this into account made them wonder if the chaos Pete was causing was his way of making a statement about his life. The constantly changing au pairs and baby-minders over the years had all spoken of Pete as a quiet adaptable boy, but now his parents were concerned that perhaps he had paid too high a price for his compliance. They went to see a child psychotherapist who agreed to work with them as a family, and also separately with Pete. Andrew said that they saw this period as a time of family crisis, and he is relieved that it didn't turn into 'Pete's crisis'. So therapy, a change of school and a change in the working lives of the parents was the solution for this family.

There are many good sites on the Internet where you can look for further help. One which stands out is ADDISS (www.addiss. co.uk) – a registered charity – which provides information, training and support for parents. They maintain a multidisciplinary assessment and treatment protocol, including education and behavioural interventions, with or without medication. They say that they try to help families find their own most appropriate approach to intervention. They also have the ADDISS Resource Centre which you can visit and which is full of information, books and a library where you can look up articles, watch videos or have a cup of tea and a chat. There is a subscription of £15 for parents to join ADDISS.

A word of warning

If you decide to go along with the drug treatment of your child, don't set your hopes too high. Is medication a band aid, a quick fix, or a much needed help for distressed children and families? Too many parents – those who approve of medication – told me that although there was improvement in the child's ability to listen and to concentrate it frequently had no affect upon many behavioural problems, especially in the demand for attention. This is another reason why medication should always be combined with therapy of some kind, since new patterns of behaviour have to be taught and learnt. So, the plus side of medication for *some* children is that it can pave the way for new parenting techniques to succeed where parents struggled before.

What if the diagnosis of ADHD is not the correct one? From many parents I heard of the diagnosis being changed again and again, often after Ritalin had failed to be of any use. What if a child is actually suffering from pathological demand avoidance syndrome (PDA) as well as ADHD, or is no more than a very, very high-spirited and energetic child? Again, this points to the necessity of an expert opinion and the importance of getting a diagnosis from someone who is properly qualified to give one, a professional experienced in looking at the *whole* picture so as to avoid a misdiagnosis. Only after a lengthy and detailed observation of a child should the diagnosis of ADHD be made.

What to keep in mind about ADHD
- ADHD is now seen as genuine disability needing treatment.
- All children show occasional behavioural problems – so don't jump too quickly to conclusions.
- It is only when some of the symptoms associated with ADHD are so pervasive and disruptive in more than one setting that the name ADHD should be given.
- Give clear and precise instructions to your child.

- Parents need support when they find ordinary parenting strategies will not work with their child.
- Medication or not? The debate rages . . .
- Some other therapies do help children with ADHD.

6

Autism

As Raun Kaufman, 26, chats fluently about his academic achievements – he was a high-school high-flyer and has a degree in biomedical ethics from an Ivy League American university – it scarcely seems credible that, at 18 months old, he was diagnosed as profoundly autistic.

(*Daily Telegraph*)

Some basic facts

Autism is known as a 'spectrum disorder,' an umbrella term used to cover a wide area of symptoms. Parents – and indeed professionals – can easily get caught up in a tangle trying to define the borderline sub-groups within the whole autistic spectrum. There is no blood test or brain scan which can pinpoint a diagnosis. According to the National Autistic Society (www.nas.org.uk) autistic spectrum disorder is estimated to affect over 520,000 people throughout the UK and, as with ADHD, it affects more boys than girls.

Over fifty years ago Leo Kanner first defined the classic autistic syndrome, but this has now been broadened to include the concept of an autistic disorder. There are three aspects to this disorder: biological, behavioural and cognitive; and discussion is ongoing about the possible multiple causes. The resulting symptoms range along a continuum from mild to severe, with a wide variation in the characteristics, so it makes a diagnosis very complicated. A child may have features producing severe disability, while at the same time showing only minor blips in another area. This is why it is important to remember that 'autistic' cannot and should not be applied to every child with just some of the symptoms, although the wider term 'within the autistic spectrum' cannot be so easily dismissed. So, although 'autism' is now more widely known about, it is still very difficult for a parent to get a diagnosis agreed upon for their child. However, an early diagnosis followed by support is of great benefit in helping a child with autism to achieve his full potential, so this is well worth striving for.

A study carried out by the Centre of Social and Communication Disorders (www.nas.org.uk/nas/elliott.htm) showed that 56 per cent of parents saw three or more professionals before getting a firm diagnosis for their child. Forty per cent of parents waited more than three years for a diagnosis, and 10 per cent waited ten years or more. The Centre was set up by the National Autistic Society in 1991. It was the first centre in the UK to provide a complete diagnostic assessment and advice service for children, adolescents and adults with social and communication disorders. However, as knowledge and understanding about autism gradually gains ground, local centres where help can be obtained towards a diagnosis are beginning to appear. If your GP does not know where to refer your child for a diagnostic assessment, the Autism Helpline (0870 600 8585) has a list of doctors and diagnostic teams with an interest in autistic spectrum disorder. And although some areas of the country are better served than others, they will put you in touch with your nearest source of help.

Indication of autism

Autism is not a mental illness, but it is a lifelong developmental disability. An autistic child looks and often acts in a 'normal' way, but he will have some odd mannerisms and may show some signs of hyperactivity. This last factor is often what decides where the diagnosis of autism, ADHD or Asperger syndrome should be made. Yet I have found that 'autism' is used indiscriminately for all three disabilities, and caution must be the watchword here. Again, this takes us into the muddy waters surrounding diagnosis. When reading about autism you may have heard about the 'triad of impairments' which need to be present: these three main areas are concerned with difficulties of communication, of social interaction and of imagination linked with an inflexibility of thought. You may have found this somewhat bewildering, so here is a list of the most prevalent features of autism:

- poor eye contact
- a lack of desire to communicate
- difficulties in relating to other people in a meaningful way, including a lack of motivation to please other people
- hypersensitivity to sound, touch, smell and visual stimuli
- difficulties with motor co-ordination
- obsessional or ritualistic behaviour
- fear of change
- need for routine
- behavioural problems
- difficulties with a regular sleep pattern
- an inability to play imaginatively
- poor attention skills.

How early are these signs likely to be apparent? Some parents told me how at even a few months, their baby did not reach out to them, nor did it want to cuddle. A reluctance to play with other children is also usually noticeable from an early age, and these babies tend to avoid eye contact more than a normal baby. These children are also likely to flap their hands and rock themselves. But, again, I must repeat that all children show different rates of maturation, so please do not jump to any hasty conclusions; any diagnosis of autism requires a *very* experienced doctor who will then follow internationally recognized criteria for a diagnosis. If your child is reluctant to play with other children, do not, I repeat *do not* make an off-the-cuff diagnosis yourself. There must always be room for the quiet and reflective child, these are still qualities to be treasured.

Even after a considered diagnosis of autistic spectrum disorder not all children will conform to the same pattern. Some autistic children will have great difficulty in using language to communicate, often with unusual patterns of speech, perhaps echoing words spoken to them, or repeating words over and over again. The hardest thing for the parents of such children is that their child will speak in order to say what it wants but will not (or cannot) use language to express feelings. Some autistic children do not develop speech at all, while others may develop speech but still have difficulty in finding words to express emotions.

The main characteristics

When autism was first identified in 1943 it was recognized that the paramount symptom was an inability to relate to people, linked with difficulties in the use of language for communication, a desire for maintaining the status quo, a fixation on some objects, with good cognitive potential. It is now widely agreed that there is a strong genetic component which plays a part in autism, and many parents will recognize that there is a family history showing this to be true. But even with this knowledge it is unfortunately not yet possible to predict which factors mean a child is likely to have autism. Over the years there has been very misleading and inaccurate information propagated about the *cause* of autism, and for a long time the finger was pointed at the mother. As a result, mothers of autistic children suffered dreadfully by being accused of being 'cold' or 'rejecting' and even 'unloving'. It has been hard to eradicate such false accusations which do not in fact bear on the cause of this disability.

As with other invisible disabilities, a child with autism looks at first sight like any other child, but often falters in areas which need communication or active social skills. This means that a child within this spectrum will have very little capacity to understand another person's point of view. An ability to empathize with others is just not there, which causes many problems in most social settings. Of course, once we are aware of this feature of autism, most of us know of adults who in our minds we are able to place within the autistic spectrum: someone who will never understand just how we are feeling, or who lacks the skill of putting himself in another's shoes for a single moment and so does not see what effect something he says is having.

Again, some children may have learning difficulties, but a significant minority have average or superior skills; assessing these may present some difficulties. Also, the use of language differs: there can be a variation from the extreme non-verbal, to a more awkward, stilted way of speaking.

Your child may not be happy with eye contact, which will have serious repercussions as he makes his way in the outside world. Other children – and many adults as well – withdraw from making contact when they, in turn, get no feedback on a social level. This pulling back may in fact be quite unconscious; it is a normal reaction when the person we are trying to talk to does not look at us, or give us any of the connecting signs others use a hundred times a day. It is surprising how much of our communication with each other is done by signals, and without these we can feel lost and, in turn, give up. Even a mother or a father can get disheartened when there is little feedback from their child, but the hard truth is that children with this difficulty need even more than their share of one-to-one attention. For them, something which develops in most of us naturally, making eye contact, just does not happen and, as a father told me, it is essential to try to teach your child the skills which do not occur spontaneously. 'We both spent time each day with David in an effort to get him to understand what we wanted him to do. We did it with perseverance and rewards and gradually David began to accept that we wanted him to make eye contact with us. From then onwards he was better with other people too. In the same way we taught him how to take turns. Believe me, it wasn't easy, but it's been worth it.'

Some case histories

Children who are autistic are often described as 'living in their own world', and at times they can be quite indifferent to others and to the feelings of others, much to the distress of their loved ones. Doreen does not like the way that children diagnosed as autistic are said to be 'out of it' so much of the time, so she felt it was her task to help 9-year-old Holly to be happy in her own space, and in this way has assisted her daughter to be content with herself and life. 'After all,' said Doreen, 'it is arrogant to suppose that Holly would be better off in "our world". It's not so fantastic, after all.'

Of course, this enclosed world may not be so extreme and you may have a child who *will* make contact with you but will only talk about what interests him or her at that particular moment. If your child's interest is, for instance, the different makes of cars, then you will probably be able to engage in a conversation with him on this topic. Eileen told me her son can even get quite animated if they go to a car park and talk about the different vehicles parked there. However, the constant repetition is very wearing for even the most sympathetic families. Eileen found that she could manipulate Adam's absorbing interest as a reward system. If he did one or two of the things expected of him – starting to get dressed, for example – then she would allow him to talk 'cars' for fifteen minutes, and she would give him her undivided attention on this topic. Another advantage is that as children get older, a subject which does hold their attention to this degree can often be channelled into a serious hobby or even a subject of research. With the Internet at everyone's fingertips today (potentially, at least) the pursuit of a special interest can reach amazing heights for older children.

Jeff told me that he had an inner feeling that something was not right with his son when he was one year old, 'although there was nothing to put my finger on at that time'. Jeff's son Tommy was a little late with his developmental milestones but this did not worry his doctor, until at the age of eighteen months he stopped using the few words he knew, ceased kissing and hugging, and became fascinated by watching the washing machine churn around and around. 'It almost seemed to happen overnight, but in fact everything did change over the course of a couple of months. We lost our boy.' Before his third birthday he was also walking on the tips of his toes and flapping his hands. 'People began to stare when we went out. Quite honestly, I was frightened out of my wits about what was happening.'

Pauline began to worry about her child when he developed a great sensitivity to certain sounds and touch. And there were occasions when he appeared not to notice her at all; he would not let her make eye contact. She did not have any worries about him until he was almost two years old, then she found it difficult to get anyone to say just what they thought was wrong with him. It was only after they moved house and a new health visitor called that the word 'autistic' was used for the first time.

'My mum said to me that she thought my baby was not developing in the right way. I was bowled over, and then began to compare him to other babies. Things got worse as he got older, he rocked and rocked himself. He seemed to comfort *himself* instead of letting me do it. As he got older he became fascinated with spinning objects and became very attached to certain inanimate things,' reported Emma. Her distress was plain to see as she remembered how hard she tried to make contact with her baby, who seemed intent on keeping his distance, even from his mother.

The activity of play is one of the areas which has made several parents aware that something was not quite right. Tara told me that she began to notice the different way her little boy played – always lining up cars and books and trains, and never wanting to play with other children. Other parents told me how their concern mounted when their child played in a repetitive, uncreative way which showed little of the imagination most children demonstrate. Tara had an assessment with an educational psychologist and was told, once again, 'Things aren't too bad.' However, after one week in mainstream school the head said that there was something seriously wrong and that her boy should be statemented.

Things then moved quickly; the paediatrician referred them to a speech therapist who diagnosed semantic pragmatic disorder (on the mild end of the autistic spectrum), and the word 'autism' was first used. Tara said that once this happened all the pieces of the jigsaw fell into place and she could see that other features, such as his extreme stubbornness and reluctance to speak to anyone outside of the immediate family, all began to make sense. She asked if I had emphasized enough to parents of children with autistic traits that, 'When I use the word "stubborn", I really do mean stubborn. It is no good "just being firm" because if faced with a child like mine however firm you are — he is just not going to do something if he doesn't want to.'

It is hard for a mother to handle this, if all the cajoling in the world will not engage the co-operation of her child. 'Stubbornness' was a word I heard over and over and over again. It seemed as if parents were telling me that there was a point beyond which their child could *not* be moved, or budged, and as the child gets older this becomes more and more of a problem. If this is coupled with an obsessional ritual it can make for desperate families.

Again, as with many other disabilities, recognition of the disorder varies tremendously. A father sent me an e-mail to say that the term autistic was unknown to him and his wife until their son was about three years old. His wife read in a magazine about autism with a description of the symptoms, and their journey along the spectrum began. They did not know any other child with this disorder. Where the family live, autism is not really known about. 'If you have money you can go to a doctor for a proper diagnosis and you can get speech therapy for your child. If you are poor you won't get any diagnosis and your child may be seen as retarded and even sent to a mental hospital.' He believes that because this reaction is rampant, most families keep their concerns to themselves. The Internet has become a lifeline, through which the family now communicate with parents in many different countries.

Help is at hand, or is it?

Even after a diagnosis there is a wide disparity about what help and support is on hand depending on where you live. I heard from parents from all over the world about the help, or lack of help, on offer.

'I hate the term autistic,' said one mother. 'I won't let it be used – I call him a special child.' From Japan I heard of the fight of one mother to get help for her son who is autistic. She told me that only now is Japanese society beginning to admit to the rights and needs of the mentally disabled, but there is little understanding or knowledge of autism. 'My 9-year-old son has had a life full of difficulties. Teachers say he is selfish but I have now found a way to speak up on his behalf.' Parents in Japan are banding together in an effort to find a stronger, clearer voice which can be heard on behalf of their children. But, it is not only in Japan that parents have fights on their hands.

A mother living in Yorkshire told me that although the school know that her son has been diagnosed as autistic, they still complain about his explosions of temper. They will not accept that for a child like Sam stress brings on fits of rage. She told me that she photocopied a list of symptoms that a child who is on the autistic spectrum disorder range is likely to exhibit, and handed out the list to all members of staff. She said that for a short while it helped. 'Then the complaints about Sam began all over again.'

'Is autism so hard to diagnose?' asked Wendy. 'We were given a run around by professionals for three years. First grommets, then tonsils, then this and then that; nothing made any difference. Eventually we had to pay for a private consultation with a neuro-paediatrician who diagnosed autism, and *then* and only then did we get some notice taken of us. But we got no help whatsoever with speech and language therapy. We had to pay for that. We also had to pay for him to go to a Montessori playgroup. We were told that "he's not bad enough for that school" and "he's too bad for this school" for him to take advantage of the facilities around here.' Wendy and Tom pushed and pushed for a statement to ensure their son would get more help but it was suggested to them that they keep him at the playgroup where he was happy. 'But we cannot afford it, my husband is a policeman and we have other kids,' said Wendy, 'but then we were told he is "too young" for this unit and then "too old" for another local unit.'

Each time there is a long wait to get an answer, 'So it all drags on and on.' She believed that many departments use delaying tactics in the hope the parents and the child will just go away. Or turn to the private sector. Wendy urged me to 'tell every parent always to hand deliver letters so they can't say it was not received. And another thing, tell parents if you don't get what you want at the beginning, you'll get nothing. Remember our kids are worth fighting for.'

Holly said that it took two years before her son was diagnosed as autistic with severe behavioural problems. He continued to get worse and harder to handle. 'Remember,' said Holly, 'the bigger they get the faster they run! I was desperate when I put him on a diet, and in a way it helped us all to get a life back. I know other children, though, where what they ate made no difference at all.'

Frank would not consider a diet for his child. As there were great problems getting him to eat at all, Frank was fearful of interfering and upsetting the balance, and certainly reluctant to stop anything which his boy would eat. Frank said: 'Parents are on their own with this, no one, *no one*, helps us. I was so naive at the beginning. I thought once there were clear indications that Charlie was autistic we would be pointed in the right direction for help.'

Other parents, too, reported being left for months between appointments. This was especially so with those families who were judged to be coping, so if you *are* managing it is important to keep this in mind. Parents who are seen to be able to pay for private treatment are often encouraged to stay in the private sector. 'I was living on benefit,' said Christine, 'but I had to find the money to pay for a speech therapist and a consultation with a homeopath somehow. I knew we couldn't wait.'

'What *do* you do', asked one mother, 'if you are told your child has only "autistic features" as we were? The professionals just washed their hands of him.' This family felt left high and dry with nowhere to turn after this diagnosis. Other families, also, would not accept a vague description because it left them unable to fight for help. Don't be afraid to ask outright whether a consultant believes your child has an autistic spectrum disorder. It may be that by speaking of autistic traits or features they are beating around the bush, and that is no help to anyone.

Mothers have told me they felt very put down by being told, 'There are children worse than yours, you know.' This makes it hard for a parent to press for help. But at what cost to the families? Parents are prepared to overcome dreadful obstacles to help their children. One family decided that the wife would take on an evening job so that she would be there for their child all day, while the husband took over the care when he got home from work. Although in one sense family life went out of the window, it did mean that their child could have the constant one-to-one attention he needed.

Pressure on the parents

There is a fine line between autism and Asperger syndrome, so that children who have poor eye contact, are hyperactive and who have no sense of danger may fall into either category. With both disabilities a frequent cause of worry is the onslaught of tantrums.

A cause of great difficulty, as you may have found, is how a parent manages a tantrum. Parents can disagree with each other about the best way forward. Do you try to appease your child, and fend off a tantrum, or will this make the child feel he can get what he wants? If you say no, your child may bang his head against the wall, or bite his own hand.

This is just one example of what can often tear a family apart. Perhaps the most widespread cause is when the parents have difficulty in agreeing about how to handle their child. What is important is consistency; if a mother has a very different approach to the father, then they are on a collision course.

Babs gave me an example. She told me that if she forgets and pulls open the curtains herself in the morning, instead of letting her son do this, 'all hell lets loose'. She has found the best way is to pull them closed again and then let him open them. Her husband disagrees with her approach, and in a similar situation will say to their son, 'Tough, I forgot.' 'Then he's off to work, and I have an upset kid for hours,' said Babs in a resentful tone. This brought about a full-blown row between these parents during our interview. Tony believes that their son has to live in the real world as well as in his own, and must learn to live alongside others as best he can.

Research carried out into depression in mothers of children with intellectual disability and/or autism (*Journal of Intellectual Disability Research*, 2001), found that mothers with children with autism had higher depression scores than mothers of those children with learning difficulties who were not diagnosed as autistic. Mothers on their own without a partner were found to be especially vulnerable to depression. This should come as no surprise because the pressure – day in and day out – on the carer of a child with a disability, any disability, can become a strain which is often too much for any parent, single or not. Marriages do break up under the pressure, and all parents of children with a hidden handicap need to be aware of this and to take every precaution they can to prevent this happening. To be the sole parent who has to deal with everything that caring for a child with special needs entails, means that even the most devoted parent is likely to crack on occasion.

From parents who are separated I heard of a major cause of aggravation. 'Nothing can make your temperature rise quicker than being told by an ex-partner that "He's okay", or, "She is fine when she is with me." ' Once again, this suggests that it is the parent who has the problem. Parents living apart number above the proportion you would expect of parents of children with a hidden disability. This is *because* the marriage has fallen apart on account of a child with a disability. So, let warning lights flash if discussions with your partner about your child end in rows, or silence. The division often comes about with a father burying himself in work or outside activities, and the mother taking over the day-to-day care of the child with special needs. It may be like the Williams family, where Jeff took on extra work to pay for the speech therapist, the occupational therapist and the private consultations needed. Sadly, this did bring about the breakup of the relationship as the couple shared less and less time together. Jeff and Helen both became silently resentful without sharing their misery; this was the last straw which broke the back of their marriage. From those parents who work together, sometimes day and night, to support and care for their child, the oft-repeated phrase is, 'We could not have done it alone – when one of us flagged the other one took up the slack.'

In his book *Breaking Autism's Barriers*, Bill Davis tells his story as a father. Anyone who is struggling to find ways of helping a child will find this book an eye-opener; it describes the difficulties this ordinary family ran into when looking for help for their son. 'From the inception of Chris' autistic symptoms, I was driven,' says the father, and the reader is left in no doubt about it. This book will be a comfort for parents in a similar situation. 'An autism diagnosis is not the end of the world. If you pay attention to your kid and learn how he operates, you'll have a wonderful life. Just give him a chance to be the best he can be.' Bill Davis is now actively involved in autism advocacy work in the US.

When at last the Stone family did get an appointment with a consultant for their child, a diagnosis of autism, query Asperger syndrome, was made. 'What happens now?' they asked. 'He would benefit from work in the communications unit we have,' was the reply. The delay in getting into this was more than a year. The Stones accept that they are fortunate for they are able to pay for a private speech therapist, and they are amazed at how quickly she has corrected many of the speech problems shown by their son.

Those parents who are most involved with their children told me that it is important to work and work and *work* at communication and that early intervention is vitally important. Maybe your child with signs of autism is placid and seemingly untroubled. It is these children above all who need us to find ways of encouraging eye contact and to develop language. 'Don't let your child just sit there staring.' 'Find places he is not scared of and take him for walks.' 'Keep a routine, but quietly introduce new experiences too.' 'Don't just wait for help from outside – it probably won't come.'

The most helpful way forward for children in the autistic spectrum disorder range is to ensure that they feel safe within a routine and in familiar surroundings. Try not to spring any surprises and do your best to maintain a constant timetable. Children feel safer when they follow a tried and tested programme.

Maxine found to her cost that if she took a marginally different route to school her son would become very distressed. So, do pay attention to detail. Something which to us may seem a very minor divergence from an everyday pattern can unsettle a child who is autistic for a considerable time.

Above all, children within this range need your time and long periods of your undivided attention – but which child does not? As all parents know, all children benefit from one-to-one time with a parent.

I was told by a mother of an adult child with very severe autism that many years ago she had to make decisions about support for the whole family. For this family the way forward was to find a weekly boarding school for their child; in time this has led to Natalie living in a community home. 'She comes home for short holidays,' said Marjorie, 'but now that we are in our seventies it is all we can manage. I am glad that all those years ago I had the foresight to find this kind of help. I know that when we are no longer here she will be cared for.' This decision was made at 'make or break time' for this couple. In similar situations the National Autistic Society can help with information about respite care.

Diet and alternative therapies

Again and again the question arose about whether a controlled diet helps a child within the autistic spectrum. There are parents who do not believe that diet has much effect. Bob is a father who would not be convinced and felt that the different programmes offered, especially the tests for allergies, were money-making enterprises aimed at desperate parents. But even parents who are sceptical about a link found that keeping a diary of foods eaten by their children revealed some surprising connections.

'For Adam it was sugar, of all things. I didn't really go for the allergy bit, but cutting out all sugar for Adam meant that he just seemed happier and a little more able to communicate with us. It can't just be chance.' I heard this from a mother who was desperate to explore any avenue. She had, in a hit-and-miss kind of way, tried to eliminate different foods for a few days at a time, and her diary pointed to some improvement in the way Adam behaved when his diet was slightly modified. 'Tell any parent to try, just try,' said Marie. 'Every little helps.'

Josh did not think that food could have all that much of an impact on his severely autistic daughter until he saw another child have a very bad allergic reaction to peanuts. It made him think that perhaps after all, 'We are what we eat, and that just maybe some foods do affect both body and brain in a way which is not always visible.' However, after putting Ali on a very strict diet he noticed no change whatsoever, except that she seemed to enjoy the extra attention which surrounded her at every meal. 'So, in a way it worked for us,' said Josh, 'but not in the way we thought it would!'

One result from research in the United States is that magnesium used with vitamin B6 helps to reduce tantrums and hyperactivity and improve speech, concentration and attention span. 'So here we go again,' said Helen. 'One more thing to try . . . but why not?'

For parents who believe that vitamin/mineral supplements do help their child, even if they are not 'the answer', there are a number of supplements available in the UK free on prescription from your GP. For more information about what is available contact the HACSG.

If you want to know more about the simple nutritional supplement LCP (long chain polyunsaturated fatty acids) found in fish oil and evening primrose oil, take a look at Dr Stordy's website (www.drstordy.com) which gives information about her work in this specialized field.

Mel tried cranial osteopathy for her daughter after reading an article about this new way to 'cure' children with autism. 'The consultation went all right, but they suggested I had to bring her every two weeks, and I was worried about the cost. It was solved for us because after the first time we could never catch my little girl in order for her to be still enough for treatment. Another dead end for us.' Cranial osteopathy originated from work of osteopath William Sutherland in the early 1900s, and is a non-invasive therapy. It is a treatment of choice for some parents for conditions such as ADD/ADHD, asthma, autism, insomnia and learning difficulties among others.

I was told about brushing therapy (neuro-dermal stimulation), which is based on the theory that many of the problems found in children with different disorders, and some developmental difficulties, can be related to an immature central nervous system. The goal of brushing therapy is to mimic the movements that should have occurred to stimulate the development of the central nervous system. It is another non-invasive treatment, but I heard from parents that it is very time consuming in an already busy schedule. 'What with medication, diet, exercises and the rest I found that brushing designated areas of the face and body several times a day with a child who won't co-operate was too much.' Further explanations and information can be found on www.bodybrushing.com.

Approaches to Autism, a pamphlet published by the NAS in 2001, is an easy-to-use guide to the many therapies which people with autism have found helpful.

From Allergy Induced Autism (www.autismmedical.com/welcome.htm) I learned that AiA was 'born' nearly twelve years ago out of an eminent Great Ormond Street doctor's observations. This UK organization now has charitable status and has gone from strength to strength. See their website where they answer questions such as, 'What can diet have to do with a condition like autism?' Part of the answer seems to be that as children develop autism they become 'picky' eaters, and often unconsciously choose a restricted diet. In addition it is believed by some parents that children who are autistic have difficulties in breaking down certain foods in the body. It is not held that dietary intervention will cure autism, but parents do swear that by watching what their child eats, it has made life easier for them and their children as *some* of the physical symptoms are relieved. There is a warning on their site that the information available from AiA should not be construed as medical advice, and that a doctor and/or registered dietician should be consulted before implementing dietary changes.

Patricia: 'My 6-year-old child who is autistic is still in nappies, so I wouldn't call it a hidden disability. But I put him on a very strict GFCF diet and a month later he is toilet trained and his speech has come on wonderfully. His rate of progress has been outstanding. I can only tell you what this diet has done for us.' (GFCF is a gluten, casein-free diet – casein is a protein found in animal's milk.) On this website there is a list of common foods unacceptable on the GFCF diet, and a list of acceptable additives together with a list of foods free from gluten, casein, monosodium glutamate and aspartame. Although, parents are still urged to check the labels as manufacturers have been known to change formulations.

'It has cost us a fortune to put Billy on a GFCF diet, but it has been well worth it. My worry is that as he gets older I won't be able to control it so well. Now when he goes to parties I can get him to take his tea in a picnic box, but I wonder how long he will want to do that.' 'My son is on a GFCF diet, and although he is only five won't accept any food from anyone else. He says, "I can't eat that, it will make me feel bad." I understood that even at such a young age he had made the connection between the way he feels and the food he eats.'

Remember the caution from AiA that any dietary intervention should be carried out in conjunction with a medical practitioner or paediatrician. Again the point is reinforced, that the autistic spectrum condition consists of a series of sub-groups, and in each sub-group there are often different bio-chemical profiles. Allergy Induced Autism has a membership fee of £10.00, and their website has a chat board where all parents can post a message. This is a helpful site giving a great deal of information about the food we eat. One entry to the AiA guest book states, 'If I got two hours sleep in any night I was grateful. I cannot begin to say just how much the diet has changed out lives.'

The National Autistic Society and understanding autism

The National Autistic Society should be the first port of call for any parent who needs to know more about autism and what help is available. The NAS was founded in 1962 and has become the UK's foremost charity for people with autism and Asperger syndrome. The NAS helpline (0870 600 8585) and their website (www.nas. org.uk) will provide answers to many questions. The society also runs training courses and conferences for professionals from all disciplines. They also have a list of clinicians known to the NAS as having an interest and expertise in developmental disorders.

A new scheme launched by the society is their Early Bird programme which is aimed at helping to support and educate parents of young children with autism. There is intensive support for three months, with lectures and home visits, and parents are videotaped applying the new skills they have learnt. The idea is to help parents to understand their child's autism and to assist them to structure their interactions to aid communication. Lack of funds prevents this scheme being widely available, but parents involved with the scheme call it 'a lifeline'.

The society offers a wide range of services including information about education, respite care and welfare benefits. They also have a very comprehensive list of helpful books. For a free catalogue call 0207 903 3595 or email publications@nas.org.uk. For example, they have a practical guide, *Teaching Young Children with Autistic Spectrum Disorders to Learn*, for parents and staff in mainstream schools and nurseries. It has a range of very helpful strategies which will be of tremendous help. Tips you may not have thought about are there, such as using a visual reminder to be quiet (a picture of a face with finger on lips). Parents have told me that they have had fun adding to this to fit in with family routine: a drawing of hands next to the lavatory is a reminder to wash hands, and a 'no entry' sign on a bedroom door has sometimes brought a few moments more of uninterrupted sleep.

Another book from the National Autistic Society is about

handling bereavement and dying, and how to help someone who is autistic to cope with the loss of a loved one. The author of *Support for the Bereaved* draws our attention to the fact, often overlooked, that because someone with autism finds any social interaction difficult it might be thought they do not form attachments to other people. If this is believed, then it may be considered that they will be insulated from grief if touched by a bereavement. However, research shows this is not always so, and many people with autism have been deeply affected by the death of someone close. Of course, all people respond differently and individually to a bereavement, but the grieving processes of people with autism are profoundly affected by their disabilities. Difficulties with communication make this whole area particularly bleak. But, you should be on the watch for delayed reaction to loss or uncertain and inappropriate responses; keep in mind that because of their disabilities of communication someone who is part of the autistic spectrum will not be able to ask for help, and so support may be needed by them to express their feelings, even to *identify* their feelings. I single out this book because I think it illuminates an area which is often totally neglected.

A parent whose daughter was eventually diagnosed as autistic nearly fifty years ago told me to urge parents to get as much help as possible. To get a diagnosis had been a nightmare. At first schizophrenia was suggested, then 'It's nothing at all', and eventually, after a private consultation, 'autism'. The day her daughter was diagnosed as autistic Dorrie was told to get in touch with a children's 'handicap society', and to consider 'putting her in a home'. That was all that was on offer in the 1950s. 'I hope things are easier for parents and children today,' she said.

Well, yes and no. The word autism is now understood to some extent by most people. But parents can still feel very isolated with their worries and concerns about their child, and about the effect on the whole family. The importance of a circle of support (professionals, parents and carers) all working together and keeping in touch with each other, and sharing observations and information, cannot be emphasized too strongly. It is when parents feel split off from the rest of us and isolated that the real anguish for families is felt. It is tragic enough to cope with the knowledge that your child has special needs, but then to find you are not able to lay your hands on something, anything, which may help is surely the unkindest cut of all.

Again the question arises, 'Do we really need a diagnosis for my child?' Hopefully, help may be more readily available once a diagnosis is made, and a diagnosis may also enable you and your child to understand more about what this disorder means. On the other hand, if you believe that your child is on the mild end of the spectrum, just understanding this may be enough.

The NAS has published a booklet entitled *Autism: Forty Years On and Still the Problem Is Understanding.* I think it is something of an indictment of our society that we should still need to be guided – or pushed – into understanding what autism means.

An important word about autism from Sara Truman, chair of a branch of the National Autistic Society, who wanted to pass on this message to parents: 'If you are worried, ask for help; the sooner the better. The problem is often convincing the professionals that there is a problem, but experts in autism agree that parents *know* when something is wrong, and should be listened to.'

Important considerations regarding autism
- Do *not* make an off-the-cuff diagnosis yourself.
- The symptoms can range from mild to severe, so the whole autistic spectrum disorder should be borne in mind.
- Don't accept a vague description from a consultant.
- If your child is autistic, try to keep to a familiar routine.
- You should be prepared to fight for the help your child needs.
- Consider the different therapies which people with autism have found helpful.
- Get all the support you can – don't be afraid to ask for help.
- Contact the National Autistic Society for information, help and support.

7

Asperger syndrome

He referred to a hole in his sock as 'a temporary loss of knitting'.
(Child with Asperger syndrome quoted on the Internet)

An unfamiliar term

Asperger syndrome, AS, is often not diagnosed until a child starts school, because that is when the difficulties in socializing are more noticeable. Before that you may have just had an uneasy feeling without being able to put your finger on what was wrong with your child. The term is used to describe people at the higher functioning end of the autistic spectrum whose main problem is difficulty in reading the signals which most of us take for granted, with the result that there are major problems in communication.

Asperger syndrome is a neurobiological disorder named after a Viennese doctor, Hans Asperger, who published a paper in 1944 describing the pattern of behaviour in a group of boys of normal language and intellectual development but who showed autistic-like behaviour in social and communication skills.

Until a few years ago 'Asperger' was a term which was seldom used, although this syndrome was first defined in the middle of the twentieth century. One advantage in using this term is that it has not yet gathered around it a heap of negative reactions in the way the names of some other invisible disabilities have. The disadvantage is that you will come up against people who have not heard of the term, and certainly do not know what it means. Parents have told me that this confusion makes it very difficult to get a diagnosis, in the UK at any rate. This means that there must be many people who have never had a formal diagnosis of Asperger syndrome and yet who have to struggle through life trying to make sense of a bewildering world.

There is no universal agreement on diagnostic criteria, but some of the signs to look for which *may* indicate AS are:

- difficulty in two-way communication
- problems with making friends
- a lack of creative play and imagination
- a monotonous voice
- a complicated vocabulary
- lack of empathy
- an apparent disregard for other people's feelings
- lack of awareness of social skills and cues
- tactlessness
- an inability to gauge personal space
- over-sensitivity to sound.

If you have already read the chapter on autism spectrum disorder (chapter 6) much of what is written there will also apply to a child with Asperger syndrome. Indeed, a child diagnosed with autism early on in life may have the diagnosis changed to Asperger syndrome at a later stage.

Problems with reading signals

However, a child with Asperger syndrome is unlikely to have learning difficulties. In addition, unlike children diagnosed as autistic, an Asperger syndrome child may not be withdrawn. Many of these children will want to make friends, but, because they find it hard to read non-verbal signals, will have difficulty in doing so. It will most likely remain a puzzle for them why they cannot fit in with other children and why at times their overtures to others are unfortunately seen as inappropriate and unwelcome. As the child grows up and begins to notice that he is often excluded or even laughed at, depression may understandably develop as a result of having Asperger syndrome. Watch out for this, especially during the adolescent years.

Asperger syndrome children will often not appreciate the give and take of a conversation or relationship, and as they find it hard to read signals, they will not be able to judge when their listener gets bored or wants to change the subject. The lack of an ability to pick up on unspoken signals can bring about many misunderstandings and issues. Jokes are likely to be difficult for them to understand, and a comment such as 'Keep that for a rainy day' will have them looking out of the window to check on the weather. The world will seem a baffling place and they will endeavour to find out why we say certain things in ways which seem complex and unnecessary. Anyone battling with AS will find making small talk a nightmare, and their blunt or plain speaking will result in people complaining of rudeness or insolence. Because of these difficulties it is important to be on the look out for teasing and baiting by other children.

A cry from one 12-year-old was typical: 'Why don't people say what they mean?' He was reacting to all those expressions so commonly understood by the rest of us: 'Hop into the car', 'She talks out of the back of her neck', 'Jump into the bath', 'She shot me an angry look', 'Don't throw the baby out with the bath water', 'Pull yourself together', and so on. To a child with Asperger syndrome it seems as if we are all talking in code, so take care to mean what you say, and avoid sarcasms and double meanings which will most likely be misunderstood and quite possibly taken literally. Children with Asperger syndrome will respond to clear instructions, but be obtuse to more subtle approaches like, 'Do you think in a moment you could possibly. . .' It will be more helpful, and avoid a situation to say, 'Bob, put your bike in the shed now.'

Other difficulties

Children with AS will often speak in a rather formal, pedantic way, and this may endear them to some grown-ups. As I heard from Lynda, 'When my son speaks he is a 6-year-old going on forty.' Children of their own age are likely to see them as 'odd' on account of their speech patterns.

Some children repeat words, either their own or something just said to them, and there is evidence that they may display signs of Tourette syndrome (chapter 16). This will show itself in facial tics or other odd movements, or making uncontrollable sounds including using socially unacceptable words or actions. If these occur, then advice from a psychiatrist should be sought.

Katie told me that when her second son was born she knew immediately that there was something different about him. She says it was hard to put her finger on what was strange except that her baby would not make eye contact, and she remembered how her other babies would search her face when breast-feeding. Both her husband and her mother laughed at her fears. However, Katie proved to be right and Jackie has grown up in 'his own special way', to use Katie's words. This means that at five he is a serious boy, a stickler for routine, and will only talk about things which interest him. He repeats facts which have caught his attention, over and over again. He is at a school which appreciates his seriousness and diligence, but he is finding playing with friends a problem. When he was invited to a birthday party recently, Jackie grew increasingly worried as the children ran about and shouted. He wanted them all to sit quietly as they do in school.

Stephanie told me that it wasn't until her son was three that there were any real worries. A referral to the local child health clinic for an in-depth check showed that his eyesight was very poor, and he had some language problems as well. It was another seven months before he could be seen by a speech and language therapist. At school the difficulties he had with socializing began to show up, and his behaviour meant that he spent more and more time removed from the class. 'We are not sure where to turn to next, but everyone at the school seems to lean towards him having Asperger's. We are waiting to have him statemented.'

Ellie considered it was a stroke of fortune to hear about Blossom House School in London, which caters for children who have a specific speech and language impairment, although they may have average or above average intellectual ability. The principal, Joanna Burgess, spoke to me of the importance of helping children early on 'before their self-esteem is shot to pieces', and how children who have difficulty in processing information need extra time and help. Children who had started in the nursery – without a previous bad mainstream school experience – were more likely to progress quickly with the support at hand. The staff-to-pupil ratio is very high, and the atmosphere in the school is one of containment, with vigilant teachers and therapists monitoring closely the different needs of each child.

The film *Rain Man* has helped more people to understand something about this condition. But nobody likes to be talked at, rather than spoken to, and this is a feature of many Asperger syndrome children and adults. In addition, all parents told me that their children were sticklers for routine and any variation brought about a very distressed child.

As a parent there are ways to help your child. You will need to teach your child some of the rules we take for granted – flexibility, sharing, co-operation and how to try to understand that actions have consequences on the feelings of others. Even try some role-playing by setting up a situation such as, 'What would you say if you saw someone wearing a strange hat?' or 'What would you say if someone gave you a present you didn't like?' or 'How do you know if someone is your friend?' Your child may need help in under-standing there is a difference between *thinking* something and saying it out loud. It is important to follow through any ideas you have. It is not enough to say, 'You mustn't say things like "you are fat".' The reply is likely to be, 'Well, he *is* fat,' and it will take some time to explain in a way a child with Asperger syndrome can comprehend that words can hurt people too. Anyone with Asperger syndrome in adult life who has to go for an interview – perhaps for a job – will need careful coaching about technique and how to 'put oneself across'.

If the condition is severe enough to want more help, and if you are in the UK, ask advice from a disablement employment officer. Through the National Austistic Society there is help for those with autistic spectrum disorders to find work, and when they have a job a key worker will support them in the workplace. Contact Prospects from the NAS (020 7833 2299).

The problems for a child may escalate as they grow into adolescence and see that friends are beginning to have relationships with the opposite sex; it is then that particular attention should be paid to explaining once again strategies which can be used. Without help a teenager may begin to withdraw from many social activities. It is a time to be particularly vigilant for signs of depression.

Jason, a little boy of seven, in a mainstream school, is causing his parents a great deal of anxiety. 'He is "in your face" from the moment he wakes until he goes to sleep,' explained his father. 'At the moment he is obsessed with facts about steam trains. He knows everything there is to know, and he talks and talks and talks about them all day every day. He hardly seems to draw breath. What that kid knows is unbelievable.' Of course this 'dedication' to a subject can, if harnessed, be turned into an asset for an adult. Computer skills have become a magnet for many Asperger syndrome children – and adults as well – and they may develop these passions into a lucrative business providing services which are on time, reliable and efficient.

Caring for a child with Asperger syndrome

A child with Asperger syndrome may be seen by outsiders to be rude or disrespectful, so it is important that adults who are involved with teaching or caring for him know that most of the behaviour is actually the result of an impairment. Although on occasion, of course, kids being kids they will inevitably be plain bad-mannered and uncivil.

Think about what you will say if you are asked to explain what Asperger syndrome is. It may be enough to say that a child who has Asperger syndrome has a neurological condition which makes it difficult for them to understand how other people are feeling, that they may be a little clumsy and develop a strong interest in one particular area. If you do not want to go into so much detail, you can simply say it is a developmental delay. Some people find the Asperger syndrome information cards, available from the NAS, very helpful.

It appears that more boys than girls are given this diagnosis, and the reason for this may be that girls are more adept at covering up, and more able to follow what is appropriate behaviour by copying what other girls are doing. Boys tend to be more disruptive and aggressive and this gets them noticed. Children with Asperger syndrome can usually attend mainstream schools, but it is important that the school responds to your child's special needs. You may have to explain the nature and effects of Asperger syndrome, and to do it on more than one occasion.

Read *Asperger United,* a self-help magazine produced by and for people with Asperger syndrome. It puts people with the condition in touch with others so that they can share information. It is free of charge to anyone with the diagnosis of Asperger syndrome who lives in the UK. Overseas readers are asked for a subscription of £6 per year to cover postage costs (email: asp.utd@nas.org.uk). A recent letter from a reader said that passing his copy of *AU* on to people who have asked about autism and what it is like has been most instructive. He also says, 'I've sat many times with tears of frustration and an overwhelming wish to be with those who live as I do. *AU* gives me that contact at times when I can't communicate.'

One website well worth looking at is OASIS (Online Asperger Syndrome Information and Support) at www.udel.edu/bkirby. asperger which is full of information for parents, professionals and kids.

Points to remember about Asperger syndrome
- You will find there are people who have not heard of this syndrome.
- There is no universal agreement on the criteria for a diagnosis.
- Because of overlapping symptoms, be knowledgeable about the whole range of the autistic spectrum disorder.
- It may not be until school age that difficulties with a child's peer group show up worrying signs.
- Children with Asperger syndrome are likely to be on the receiving end of bullying.
- Children with Asperger syndrome respond to clear instructions.
- Evolve a routine to keep down your child's anxiety level.
- Watch out for signs of depression, especially in older children with Asperger syndrome.

8

ADD
(attention deficit disorder)

The human brain has a mind of its own.
(Joseph Heller, *God Knows*)

Diagnosing ADD

ADD is not new, so a report in the medical journal *The Lancet* in 1902 describing a doctor's early observation of a child with all the signs of ADD makes interesting reading:

> Boy, aged six years was unable to keep his attention to a game for more than a very short time, and the failure of attention was very noticeable at school, with the result that in some cases the child was backward in school attainments, although in manner and conversation he appeared as bright and intelligent as any child should be.

This description shows real insight, since a century ago ADD had not been identified; it is only now that ADD as a disorder is becoming more widely recognized.

ADD (ATTENTION DEFICIT DISORDER)

There is growing recognition of this disability, especially when a child's constant inattention makes parents and teachers wild with frustration. It appears to have a bio-neurological basis, and brain scans of people with ADD give evidence of this, but they do not help with a diagnosis. ADD occurs in varying degrees of severity and is not something that someone can just outgrow. A mild case can be helped by understanding the condition and by introducing strategies to cope with the behaviour it produces; even severe conditions can be helped with appropriate support. ADD always begins in childhood, although there are many adults with ADD, but, of course, this would not have been recognized as a condition when they were young.

The problem is not so much lack of attention and concentration – indeed someone with ADD may be able to focus on a task for long periods of time – but there is likely to be a problem with *regulating* attention when needed, and then holding that attention to the task in hand. Again, more boys than girls are diagnosed as having ADD.

Children with mild ADD are often not regarded as having a disability. If they are quiet and well behaved children, not hyperactive and do not create problems for others in the same way as a child with ADHD does, their disability may go unrecognized for some time. They may just coast along, but it is more than likely that they will soon find themselves 'in trouble' at school for daydreaming or not seeming to concentrate and for failing to complete tasks.

According to the Milton Keynes ADD/ADHD Support site (www.mk-adhd.org.uk), 40 per cent of all children with ADD have at least one parent with the same condition, although it may never have been diagnosed. Also, there is a strong possibility that as many as 30 per cent will have a sibling showing signs of ADD. Although acceptance of attention deficit disorder as a bio-neurological condition has gained ground, there are still people who do not believe a diagnosis of ADD should be made *except in the most extreme cases* where impulsiveness is also prevalent. It is a very complex condition to diagnose, and although there will be some similarities between children with ADD there will also be major differences. And once again you need to remember, it is only when the difficulties persist that you should begin to be concerned and look for a diagnosis. However, for a child with mild ADD there are strategies to help him.

The signs which taken together suggest that a child has ADD are when he:

- has difficulty in regulating attention
- is disorganized
- gives the impression of being overwhelmed
- is creative
- is imaginative
- is impulsive
- makes careless mistakes
- seems not to listen when spoken to
- is forgetful
- is easily distracted
- has difficulty in sustaining relationships
- loses things
- has low self-esteem
- shows signs of other conditions – learning difficulties, anxiety, depression and Oppositional Defiant Disorder.

Children who exhibit a more obvious disability of ADD show signs also of disorganization, procrastination and chaos. However, although the impulsiveness of a child with ADD may create difficulties, it is usually problems with poor attention which bring this disorder to the fore.

A child may have severe difficulties in screening out background noises, and therefore be unable to concentrate on the task at hand if he is in a noisy classroom, hears a baby crying or if there is a noise in the street outside. Hopefully our understanding of this condition is growing all the time and will result in a more sympathetic approach to those affected by the condition.

Is it a disability?

I heard from parents who had been called into their child's school and were shocked to hear ADD being spoken about for the first time. As some children with ADD find it difficult at times to focus for lengthy periods, they may appear lazy or give the impression of not trying hard enough. In a busy classroom setting it is all too easy to overlook the child who is struggling with this invisible disability. But *is* it a disability? Many professionals do not believe it is, and instead describe these children as having above average creativity and imagination. Often routine work at school does not engage their attention, and the daydreaming begins.

I heard also from a child psychotherapist who cast doubts on the growing number of children said to have ADD. She believes that many children are over-stimulated or over-stressed and therefore simply 'cut off' at times. Her words of caution are for parents to make sure that their child is simply not overloaded in this busy world and with a way of shutting down when things get too much. She said she always asks a parent to check: 'Does your child have time everyday just to play? Does your child ever have time to be on his own without the TV on or a walkman clamped to his ear? Is there anything happening in the family which could be distressing this child?'

Parents who have come up against it

Anthea: 'We have a quiet thoughtful little girl, and we went wild with anger when we were told she has a problem. We changed her school at once and she is much more involved with the imaginative work they do. Her new teacher keeps a look out and if Susie starts to gaze out of the window she makes sure that her attention is recaptured. I shudder to think what would have happened to Susie if we had left her at her old school.' Anthea also told me that a friend of hers had a child, Richard, at this school and a diagnosis had been made of ADHD because 'he is too energetic'. Are schools now less tolerant of children who do not fit the norm? Do we want all our children to be 'middle of the road'? Is there any room at all for a child like Susie who is quiet and needs, from time to time, to be drawn into class-work, or for a boy like Richard who needs to be given additional tasks to use up his enormous amount of energy? A wise parent or teacher, if they have the time and understanding, will find ways of harnessing this surplus energy in an overactive child.

Parents are often at their wits' end to know if inattention and a certain vagueness is a real disability or not. This may cause problems if there are times when a child concentrates very well, especially in a one-to-one situation. It is often the *selective* attention which many children have that gets them into big trouble at school. It can bring about such comments as, 'You see, you can do it when you try,' whereas a child may have very little control in this direction at all.

Thomas: 'I know my kid has a problem, but it's hard to keep my patience sometimes. Tell me, is this ADD a disability, or do I just have a child who needs a bit more help to pay attention to detail?' A common enough enquiry. And just as with a child with AAP (auditory attention problem), there are strategies which can help; making sure a child has heard and *taken in* what is being said to him is one of the most important. It may be hard going to tell your child over and over again something which he needs to concentrate on and remember, but it will be worth it. You shouldn't take it for granted that your child's attention has been focused upon you and what you are saying. Make sure it has, and this will prevent those scenes which can rapidly develop into a parent shouting, 'I told you so,' or, 'Don't you ever listen to what I am saying?' And remember that praise for things done and carried out as they should be, always goes down well.

Medication and other strategies

When a child's inattention is continually evident at home and at school, the issue begins to get complicated and this is where the staff may decide to speak with the parents. A child may find himself in big trouble at school for making careless mistakes, appearing not to listen, and general lack of concentration. Medication may be suggested, but this is certainly *not* the treatment of choice for many parents, even after an informed diagnosis of ADD. But if this is your decision, it is as well not to expect miracles.

Parents who did opt for medication have told me that there was an improvement in the ability to concentrate but that where there were accompanying temper tantrums and anti-social behaviour, these symptoms often persisted.

David Pentecost, a family therapist who has written *Parenting the ADD Child*, has developed some practical strategies for managing behavioural problems in children diagnosed with ADD. His ADDapt programme stands for 'ADD alternative parenting techniques' and is a guide for parents on how to deal with the disruptive behaviour patterns common to *some* children. He believes that ADD can be a parenting nightmare, and that parents need extra special skills to manage the behaviour. According to Pentecost the golden rule is 'Be consistent', and this has been reinforced by parents who have told me that they believe that their children find any mixed messages confusing and upsetting. (This is so, too, with children with other special needs, especially for kids with autism and other developmental delays.)

There is a correlation between learning difficulties, such as dyslexia, and ADD. And as with all these disorders those who are on the mild end of the spectrum can be helped with strategies and one-to-one support. ADD will not go away as a child grows up: but adults frequently find ways of managing their difficulties and can cope, for example, with their impulsive behaviour by being aware of its consequences. Adults will have found, too, that stress and other factors can have an effect upon the way they feel and behave and will have learnt to avoid certain situations.

Brian told me what it was like to be a child with ADD characteristics over thirty years ago. 'I never quite knew what was going on. There were times when I felt clued in, and then others when I was really off somewhere in my head. I never knew which way it would be.' Even so, he did not believe he had a handicap or disability and can see in his own daughter the kind of fey behaviour he remembers from his own childhood. 'I just make sure that she is as prepared for the day as she can be,' he said. 'Now she is a little older I have talked to her about the situation. I have shown her how to make lists of things she has to do and remember, to make goals for herself, and to pepper her room with Post-it stickers to remind her to do things. She is doing okay, considering.' He told me he had not told the school because he believed that there would be little sympathy, and any undue attention makes Lilly stressed and more likely to 'cut-off' from the world.

Brian also believed that the anxiety and low self-esteem felt by many people with even mild ADD is because of the intolerant attitude of others. In this busy world it seems as if we are all expected to jump to it, and anyone who is lagging behind is seen as annoying and irritating.

'Henry does half of his homework, then starts to fiddle around. It seems he goes off the boil,' said Derek. I was told that this can often end with the whole family screaming at each other as they try to get Henry to buck up and get finished. The school came up with the answer: if Henry has not finished his homework in the given time, then he should send in his work uncompleted. The suggestion of a clock in front of Henry helped him to plan his time, a little, and the frustration of trying to chivvy him into finishing a set piece of work came to an end. 'It was hard for me to understand that Henry didn't work at the efficient speed that I do,' said Derek. This family learnt the hard way that all the explaining in the world will not prevent someone with ADD procrastinating in a manner likely to enrage onlookers – unless they understand what is happening.

Both Brian and Derek give strong reminders of the point I have tried to reinforce again and again – that all children are different, they mature at different rates, and even if your child seems more forgetful than others it may be in your best interest to accept that that is how he is. Whoever said that we have to be firing on all cylinders at all times? By all means help with some strategies as Brian has suggested, but unless the symptoms are very severe just make sure your child has the support needed, and the extra time that it will take to get dressed or to do homework. It often helps if you can make a setting for homework where there are few distractions, and if the school is informed they too may find that by seating your child in a quieter spot he can be helped a great deal with concentration. Someone who has ADD will probably not pay enough attention to social signals, so teach your child to recognize indicators that other people are sending out. By being 'distracted' a child may miss a great deal of what is going on, and this is where you can aid him by helping him recognize the clues.

If being impulsive is a problem for your child, try to make him understand what this means, and how difficult his behaviour can be for other people. Try to help your child identify situations where he might act in an impulsive way. A good idea is to role-play situations with him where he needs to pick up signals from you before blurting something out. Anger and impulsivity often go hand in hand, so the more rapport you and your child have, the less likely is he to fly off the handle. Remember, too, that an explosion may come from fear. Ronnie: 'I remember after I had been off dreaming I would come to with a start, not really knowing what people were talking about and would sometimes get scared and make a fuss about nothing at all just to show myself that I was back!'

Justin: 'All my report cards showed I was intelligent but "didn't pay attention". I wish someone had explained to me what was happening.' So talk to your child and try to understand if he is worried about any 'missing' time, and see what strategies you can work out together. Adolescents are more able to make use of beepers and computers to remind them of places where they should be and at what time.

If we look around us we are very likely to see people who show signs of ADD, although we may regard them as 'vague' or 'dreamy' and even at times uncaring. Maybe they cannot connect with the way others are feeling, or they do not realize the effect something they do or say will have on another person. Again, it may not be inattention that we notice in an adult, but rather a determined way of concentrating on a task which appeals to them. This trait is what makes it all the more puzzling when other significant things are forgotten or disregarded. Life with ADD, for both adults and children, can at times be a torment of trying to guess what is going on and to make up for what may have been missed.

Sarah: 'If only we had been able to *see* there was something wrong with Anthea. Before we knew about ADD we just thought she was naughty. Even our doctor told us that it must be *me*, and that I was "worrying because I wasn't accepting the limits my child could achieve". But I am still not convinced it is a disability – a problem yes, but not a disability.'

A very helpful and informative website to visit is www.ADD helpline.org.

Helpful hints about your child with ADD

- ADD always begins in childhood and occurs in varying degrees of severity.
- This is a hidden disability which can be overlooked if a child is 'quiet' or 'well behaved'.
- A child may show *selective* attention which means there can be difficulty in *regulating* attention when needed and concentrating on a task.
- A child with ADD may find himself in trouble at school for daydreaming.
- Strategies which will help your child with mild ADD:
  - let him study where it is peaceful and where there are no distractions;
  - make sure he has truly understood and taken in any instructions;
  - make sure he is not overloaded or over-stimulated;
  - be consistent and do not give him mixed messages which confuse him;
  - watch out for signs that your child is 'distracted' or 'impulsive'.
- Talk to your child and try to explain what you think is happening, and why.

9

Being gifted

In short, gifted kids need a parent advocate. That advocate is you.
(Joan Franklin Smutny, *Stand Up for Your Gifted Child*)

Children who are different

This is a tricky area as it is difficult to define just what is meant by 'gifted'. We all gasp at the news that a 5-year-old boy has passed his GCSE in maths and the media give him star treatment for a while. But, although he may be a mathematical genius, is he up to standard in everything else, and what is he like emotionally? A child can be very able in one area but not in others. The National Foundation for Gifted and Creative Children (www.nfgcc.org) include the following features in their criteria for diagnosis of a gifted child:

- excellent memory
- extensive vocabulary
- fast learner
- good at problem solving
- very good at puzzles, etc.
- wide range of interests

- keen observer
- perfectionist
- high sensitivity
- excessive amounts of energy
- easily bored with an apparent short attention span
- an inability to sit still unless absorbed in something of his own interest.

Although one's initial picture of a child who is 'gifted' is of a student who sails through school with excellent marks and who has perfect social skills, this may be far from the truth. Often these children feel disadvantaged by not being understood, and they are aware that they are 'different' and 'not on the same wavelength' as their peers. These children may also find it difficult to express their feelings and are inclined to develop a fear of failure. The NFGCC found that children they tested exhibited a high IQ, but they often showed 'frozen' creativity as well.

A child may be 'bright' but not gifted: the definition depends upon the degree of ability. In her book *Stand Up for Your Gifted Child* Joan Franklin Smutny – the founder of the Center for Gifted Children at National-Louis University in the US – differentiates between the two. For her the bright child 'knows the answers, and is interested. The gifted child *asks* the questions, and is extremely curious.' It is interesting to note, too, that her checklist for the traits that a gifted child displays includes some of the signs we have seen earlier in other diagnoses: he can 'multitask' (concentrate on two or three activities at once), talk like an adult, resist conforming, has trouble sitting still, devotes time to building up elaborate collections of ephemera or other objects about which he is passionate, tends to rebel against what's routine or predictable and he demonstrates high energy. Although these characteristics may be included in other disabilities, note that her list includes additional features which do *not* appear in the ADD/ADHD diagnosis. Joan Franklin Smutny also warns about the way gifted children are especially susceptible to social pressures and the problems which can arise by them 'feeling different'.

Bob told me that his son Kevin never seemed to have the same interests as other children of his age. Kevin always dismissed the latest fads and crazes that enthralled the others as 'kids' stuff'. And they in turn called Kevin a 'boff' and 'stuck up'. 'He was okay in one sense with children older than himself, but only in some respects. He was obviously brainy, but emotionally still very much younger. He just didn't fit in anywhere.'

Of course, we all know children who seem to be able to read at a very early age and who fly through the school curriculum with ease. But there can be a downside too. A child who is very bright may all the same have difficulties with some concepts; he may have out-standing abilities in abstract reasoning, yet be unable to process the information. The consequence of this is that gifted children are often at risk of being diagnosed as ADD. However, the opposite can happen too. Brian told me that his son has all the symptoms of a child with ADHD, but because he has an exceptionally high IQ no one will confirm the diagnosis. Brian said life is often a torture for his son, who devours information but at the same time is unable to sit still.

Consider the difficulty for some children who are cleverer than average but find at an early age they can easily become bored or restless. Quite often these children have a high level of energy, and if this is not directed into a creative channel it may be seized upon as one of the indications that the child has a disability. Ofsted, the school inspectorate in the UK, believes that gifted children are being neglected by state schools. This government watchdog has reported that schools need to do more to increase the pace for bright pupils. This may surprise you, but the irony is that pupils who are under-achieving because they are not sufficiently stimulated are often mistaken for low-ability candidates.

It is necessary to tailor the learning of a gifted child to meet his needs *before* he becomes disinterested and acts out with unruly behaviour. Of course, it is not only the gifted child who may get bored at school; bright pupils under-perform if they are not being stimulated enough by the curriculum and find the pace of learning too slow. This can lead to a child misbehaving or just opting out, with the risk of a diagnosis of ADHD or ADD. Indeed, many parents support the view that quite frequently a child diagnosed with ADHD is a bored child. It is important that a child who gets easily impatient and has a low tolerance for detail should be properly evaluated, especially if he is considered gifted

Gifted children have special needs too

Being gifted can also be a disadvantage, since many gifted children learn to cover up the fact that they find most things very easy to learn. They become expert at masking the gaps in their understanding, which can lead to difficulties later with their studies. And this in turn may make them *underachieve* causing frustration and bad behaviour.

A study in 2001 by Professor Joan Freeman, a psychologist at Middlesex University, found that more of those *referred to* as 'gifted' grew up to be introverted and unhappy than those pupils of the same ability who were not saddled with the tag. She believes it puts an unnecessary burden on the children who cannot cope with the expectations heaped on them at a young age. The children who were not labelled as such tended to live happier lives. It is thought-provoking to read that Professor Freeman found 'the ones labelled gifted had more problems at home, with a higher rate of divorce, and unhappiness at school about being labelled gifted'. She reminds us that being gifted does not mean emotionally distressed, but refers to normal people with special gifts. The media also likes to seize upon stories of children known as 'troubled geniuses', who although 'gifted' enough to be at Oxbridge when still at primary school age then become estranged from their families. Remember that children do not like to be seen as different in any way – even with a label that to the rest of us may seem to be an advantage.

After speaking with families I was left in no doubt that many gifted children have special needs too which are not always recognized or catered for. The Government in the UK has recently announced that £60 million has been earmarked to pilot an academy for gifted and talented children. There will be special emphasis on mentoring for the children, additional support for parents and teachers, and the targeting of deprived areas. This project has, predictably, brought about mixed reactions from teachers and parents. Some teachers believe that by picking out the brightest pupils the rest will be demoralized, but on the other hand it is felt to be wrong if bright children have to go through school at the pace of the national average. The director of the centre for research and assessment at the Institute of Education has spoken wisely: 'The tests will label the children as clever but what happens after that? . . . Maybe we have just gone testing mad.'

What is often overlooked is that a child may be gifted *and* have learning difficulties. There are children who are highly creative and inventive when not in a learning situation, whose approach to what is going on in class may not fit in with what the teacher expects. A child may have to struggle to remember facts or to produce the kind of work that his class teacher wants. The difficulty may lie in processing the information. If in these circumstances it can be recognized that a child is having a problem, something as simple as giving him extended time to complete a task can be tremendously helpful. If a gifted child has problems with written language his promise and skills may be overlooked; this is when a clever child may just give up. So if your child shows signs of dyslexia or dysgraphia (problems with writing) try to ensure they have help, especially with tests. Some schools now permit the use of computers to make it easier for children who otherwise would have struggled to organize and edit their work.

A mother interviewed by the *Daily Telegraph* said that her child at eighteen months old could count to twenty and recite the alphabet. When he began school, 'They were fantastic,' and arranged for him to do advanced number work. However, by the time he was seven they said they could do no more for him and suggested the parents should consider private education. So, one more child with special needs found the system lacking.

I recommend you visit www.giftedmonthly.com. This is a UK site which addresses the everyday needs and concerns of parents with gifted children and has a monthly newsletter. You will find extensive information, and you can visit the 'gifted community' where parents can meet or answer each other's questions.

History has some encouraging examples for us to take notice of: Einstein was four years old before he could speak and seven years old before he could read. A newspaper editor fired Walt Disney because he had 'no good ideas', Winston Churchill failed his school examinations, and Thomas Edison was told by a teacher he was too stupid to learn anything. Gifts may lie dormant for years – encouraging news for parents if they are struggling with a child who cannot understand certain basic principles.

> *Children who are gifted may also show signs of:*
> * uneven skills;
> * becoming distressed by feeling 'different' to their peers and not fitting in with their age group;
> * Getting easily bored;
> * having difficulty in sitting still unless they are absorbed in a subject or hobby;
> * having their own way of wanting to learn;
> * learning difficulties.

10

PDA (pathological demand avoidance syndrome)

Man often thinks he is in control when he is being controlled;
while his mind is urging him in one direction his heart is dragging
him in another, though he knows it not.

(La Rochefoucauld, *Maxims*)

A new syndrome

PDA is a condition which was first identified and named by Professor Elizabeth Newson in the 1980s. It is still not officially recognized in the diagnostic manuals, but it is now diagnosed in many paediatric departments. Symptoms are classed as a pervasive developmental disorder related to, but separate from, the autistic spectrum. Before recognition of this syndrome children would probably have been diagnosed as having 'atypical autism', 'atypical Asperger syndrome' or 'pervasive developmental disorder not otherwise specified'. Fifty per cent of children with PDA are girls, according to Professor Newson's research (based on a sample of one hundred).

165

Symptoms of this hard to diagnose disability include:

- obsessional demand avoidance (100 per cent)
- socially manipulative behaviour (100 per cent)
- overactive imagination with uncertainty between reality and fantasy
- lack of boundaries
- impulsiveness, lability of mood
- display of extremes of emotion with nothing 'in between'
- diversionary tactics – especially distraction
- bargaining (but the child seldom keeps his or her bargain)
- withdrawing into role-play
- talking non-stop
- screaming, kicking and lashing out
- non-cooperation.

(More detailed descriptions are available from the Early Years Diagnostic Centre, telephone 01623 490879.)

A child with PDA may have been very passive as a baby, and although he may have missed some of the early milestones, it is only when the outside world begins to make demands that problems begin to show. And although, unlike a child with Asperger syndrome, he may appear to be superficially socially skilled, he will have problems with social communication of a different kind. Someone with PDA will usually have good eye contact, which can be quite threatening at times, particularly when this is used to manipulate others socially.

One characteristic of many individuals with PDA is that they are obsessive with *people* not things, and need to feel they are in complete control of every situation. They react in a pathological manner to ordinary demands and requests made to them. This may be either by verbal or physical distraction, since anyone with PDA becomes an expert in avoidance tactics.

Even very young children become skilled in tactics to make sure they remain in command of every situation. Sara: 'My child over-whelms me with words. If I make the mildest suggestion to him he turns on me and I feel I am drowning.' Sara's husband agreed, and added, 'If we just let him get on with things by himself, he's okay, but once the focus is on him he goes wild and will go to any length to stop us asking him to do anything at all. Now we understand that it is underlying fear we can be more understanding, unlike the rest of the world who see him as rude and naughty with a "don't care" attitude.'

What many people find difficult to believe is that it is often the child's inability to deal with what he perceives as stress, even with the ordinary everyday things we all do, which makes him lash out. If the child is uncertain about whether he will accede to a demand his anxiety level rises in a way unlikely to elicit much sympathy or understanding. Especially as on one level he seems socially adept with an ability to mask his difficulties, but then suddenly disregards everyone else's feelings.

Children with PDA often have a highly developed skill of mimicry, and so by copying how others behave they may appear to fit into the curriculum of a mainstream school. Angela: 'My son has been diagnosed with PDA. I understand it now, but before I did I could never work out why he would come home from school one day and sound and behave just like one of his friends, or teachers.' Other PDA parents told me that their children can get 'stuck' in acting out different roles, because they find it hard to know the difference between fact and fiction. Mainstream school with strong support is preferable where possible, because the peer models are better, but precautions against bullying are needed because these children are easily 'set up'.

Where to find help

The website of the Pathological Demand Avoidance Syndrome Contact Group (www.pdacontact.org.uk) is a mine of information. The site's main role is to offer telephone support to parents and children with PDA, and also advice for anyone living or working with a child or adult diagnosed with PDA. Details of their annual conference is given on the website and most of the information on the site is derived from the research of Professor Elizabeth Newson. Contact her centre, the Early Years Diagnostic Centre, Nottingham, for support and information, advice and diagnosis, and for their 'Educational and Handling Guidelines'.

Jan Seaborne, who is a mother of a child with PDA, runs the PDA Contact Group with the support of other parents in a similar situation. The group offers a 'listening ear, support and information about the condition'. The group is affiliated to Contact a Family and is hoping to obtain registered charity status. Any parent battling for a diagnosis will find help here; the email address is jan@pda contact.org.uk. Jan also believes in the efficacy of massage to help children with many invisible disorders. She recommends a visit to the International Association of Infant Massage (www.iaim.org.uk) to find out more.

Donna, who has a child diagnosed with PDA, says, 'My son has excellent support at school with a "wonderful" learning support assistant, who uses the "personality based approach". She uses lots of humour and variation. My son knows her boundaries, but will still pathologically test them, and she know this.' Sadly, this kind of support is not there for all parents and their children who are often excluded from school.

'My boy is now calmer at home,' although Donna can recognize the warning signs if he is anxious about something. 'He has what I term the "camouflage effect". He has learnt a way of being which is to perform a bare minimum in order to keep the demands on him low. When the demands increase then so does his anxiety and he no longer has the ability to camouflage. He camouflages if he is coping and resorts to shock tactics if anxious or not coping.'

Some parents have tried prescribed medication, but they report there is only short-term relief.

Of all the hidden disabilities PDA is one of the hardest for parents to manage; one reason being that it is still not recognized by many professionals. Typical comments from parents are: 'No negotiation about anything ever', 'I thought I would go mad with his behaviour', 'I am at my wits' end to know what to do – everyone says it is the parents' fault', 'At nursery they said there was nothing wrong with him – he was just hard to handle. I should say so!'

Strategies to help with PDA
- Try to understand the fear and panic behind the symptoms.
- Treat tantrums as a panic attack.
- Avoid confrontation, use *indirect* requests.
- Handle carefully and, above all, avoid stressful situations.
- Accept that the usual praise/reward/punishment/parental strategies will not work with a child with PDA.

11

Dyspraxia

The term dyspraxia comes from the word praxis, which means 'doing, acting'.
Dyspraxia affects the planning of what to do and how to do it.

(Dyspraxia Foundation website)

What is dyspraxia?

Dyspraxia or 'developmental dyspraxia', as it is often called, is a descriptive term for the condition of those children who have co-ordination difficulties – and the range of these difficulties can be extensive. There is a strong overlap between dyspraxia and dyslexia and symptoms often interconnect. The Dyspraxia Foundation – their website address is www.dyspraxiafoundation.org.uk – defines dyspraxia as 'an impairment or immaturity of the organization of movement. Associated with this there may be problems of language, perception and thought.' Dyspraxia is one of the more obviously hidden disabilities and this means that parents are uncertain for some time just *what* is not quite right in the development of their child. You will probably have found that many people do not know what the term 'dyspraxia' means; it is a condition which is often not diagnosed at all. Yet dyspraxia affects up to one in twenty children with boys identified four times as frequently as girls. The fact is that someone who is dyspraxic does not necesarily seem to have a disability at first glance, but the problems which stem from this disability can be considerable.

Dyspraxia is an immaturity of the brain resulting in messages not being clearly transmitted to the body. Not all the problems caused by dyspraxia will be experienced by everyone with the disability, and by no means to the same degree, so do keep this in mind. Some dyspraxic children will have other learning difficulties as well, while some will be at the other end of the spectrum and have above-average intelligence.

According to the Dyspraxia Foundation these are some of the problems caused by dyspraxia:

- clumsiness
- communication impairment
- poor posture
- walking awkwardly
- confusion about which hand to use
- difficulty in throwing a ball
- sensitive to touch
- finding some clothes uncomfortable
- poor short-term memory, often forgetting tasks learnt the previous day
- poor body awareness
- reading and writing difficulties
- inability to hold a pen or pencil properly
- poor sense of direction
- inability to hop, skip or ride a bike
- slow to learn to dress or feed on one's own
- inability to answer simple questions even though knowing the answers
- speech problems – slow to learn to speak, or speech may be incoherent
- prone to phobias or obsessive behaviour
- exhibiting impatience

- intolerance of having hair or teeth brushed, nails or hair cut and resistance to band-aids as too uncomfortable to wear.

Not everyone who is dyspraxic will exhibit these characteristics, so I urge parents to take careful note of this. Please do not jump to conclusions just because your child does not like having his hair cut! I don't know of any 3-year-old boy who does. Also, if you already have one child you will know there is a great variation in the age at which children willingly dress themselves. But like other invisible disabilities it is when a cluster of problems make themselves noticed that it may be time to consider just what is happening, or not happening, to your child.

Some case histories

It is often clumsiness and poor balance, together with walking awkwardly, which are the first signs to worry a parent. Indeed for some time dyspraxia was often called 'clumsy child syndrome'. For Anthea, her worries began when her baby was slow to move and obviously did not enjoy 'getting going' as most babies do. Once her son was mobile there was a constant stream of accidents, and it was these which sent her looking for an answer to what was wrong. She became worried about Joe's co-ordination, and when it was agreed that he had poor gross motor movements he was referred to a physiotherapist and then to an occupational therapist. Joe was also slow to speak, and eventually a dual diagnosis of dyspraxia/dyslexia was made. However, before the diagnosis was pronounced Anthea went through the agony shared by so many parents of believing that somehow her poor parenting was to blame. She told me that the level of guilt she felt was indescribable, and only by seeing a psychotherapist for some time could she begin to accept that her son had a disability *through no fault of hers*. Anthea began to remember that other people in the family had shown some signs of poor co-ordination, and she recalled that at school she had found it impossible to learn her tables and even today her writing is considered 'sloppy'.

Patti said that it was not until her son was seven that she could understand and accept that he had a problem. Her mother told her that as a child Patti herself had been a late starter, and not to fuss about Stan who was slow to talk clearly and moved in an awkward way. 'I tried to get help, but I was told it was two years' wait to get an appointment with a physio, and two to three years to see an educational psychologist.' Eventually, Patti and her husband decided to pay for a consultation, and it was then that dyspraxia was diagnosed. 'We had never heard the word before.' Again, these parents reported that they had no support. To add to their dismay they saw signs that other parents did not really want their children to play with Stan. 'You would think he had something which was catching,' said Patti.

She was later told by another parent that there had been fears in the nursery that the other children would copy the way Stan spoke and walked, and so this was why they had not invited Stan to play. 'Once he could talk more clearly other mothers showed their surprise with comments like, "Oh, Stan is really quite bright then." That really, really hurt.'

Lynda was in America when she first began to worry about her little boy. She found help was available immediately, and the school David went to had a 'buddy' support system going. This meant that an established mother would keep an eye on a new mother and child, and so Lynda found that she and her son were well supported. Coming back to the UK Lynda discovered that things were very different. Although she felt some lip-service was paid to her boy at school, the condition of dyspraxia was not taken on board, and she was told that many of the staff considered it just one more 'crazy American idea'. Lynda felt there was no understanding or support from other mothers, and that David was ostracized and his behaviour often mistaken for 'not being brought up properly'. Laurie told me, too, that when he had asked at his son's nursery whether Bobby might be dyspraxic, he had received the frosty reply, 'Oh, why do all parents want a medical label on something their child is having a problem with. He is an ungainly child, and will probably grow out of it.'

To have a child who is dyspraxic can put a heavy burden on parents, as this is a disability which is difficult to define and goes hand in hand with little understanding about the problems parents and children face. For a parent there are often years of see-saw uncertainty: 'There is something wrong.' 'No there isn't.' 'Oh yes, I am afraid there is.'

'Did you know there is a high proportion of men in prison who are dyspraxic and/or dyslexic?' asked James. 'I wasn't surprised to read that, because I know the fight I had on my hands to get help for my boy. Any parent not able to gen up on what it might be must really be at sea.' James is right, and there are parents who will not accept that their child is struggling at all. This does not help because it is only by acknowledging the effort shown by their child to overcome his difficulties that they can provide the support he needs. If the symptoms are ignored, the consequences can be profoundly damaging.

Playing ball and hopping are among the difficulties these children experience. And this is where concerned parents are often told by friends and other parents that they are fussing about nothing, and that all children catch up in the end. *And many children do*. However, the parents themselves cannot so easily dismiss those early feelings of apprehension as they see their child unable to skip and ride a bike with friends.

Anna told me that when she mentioned to her mother-in-law that she was concerned about Daniel's development, her mother-in-law flew into a rage and told her to stop picking holes and to let Daniel develop at his own pace. When Anna mentioned her worry about dyspraxia this only seemed to add fuel to the fire. 'You are caught up by the media to find a fashionable label for Daniel – DON'T DO IT. He is a lovely little boy and you will turn him into a DISABLED child.' Anna said this was one of her lowest moments as she continued to be apprehensive every time she watched Daniel at play. Only that morning she had seen him trying to copy his friends who were drawing. The fact that he found it awkward to hold a pencil was obvious, and Anna couldn't help but compare him to the other kids of the same age or even younger.

Anna's concern – and her husband's – about whether to get an assessment for Daniel really brought about a family rift. In fact both sets of grandparents were violently opposed to drawing attention to any of the increasing number of things which Daniel was not able to do. Meanwhile, as other children began to dress and feed themselves, Daniel did not. However, when he *was* interested in something, like cars, she suddenly saw a boy who could organize and categorize the different colours and makes very efficiently. 'But,' said Anna, 'every time I stopped worrying, something else would happen.' She noticed that when they were out shopping Daniel had a very poor sense of danger or direction, even when in a familiar setting, and would often just wander off and get lost.

Anna felt she had to look outside the family for support and a friend recommended a nursery which had an interest in children with special needs. She said she liked the attitude of the staff, and they were particularly vigilant about safety. Daniel is more comfortable playing with younger children now, and although this does not present a problem in the five to seven age group, Anna fears that it will cause problems later on. Meanwhile, she is searching for a school which will have special awareness of a child with dyspraxia – although Daniel has not been 'officially' diagnosed as such up to this moment. Anna told me that she was becoming more confused about what is wrong with Daniel. At four years old Daniel has already found ways of avoiding tasks he knows he would find difficult.

She had spoken to another mother who has a son diagnosed as autistic, and hearing about 9-year-old Brian made Anna wonder if she should pursue that avenue. Again, this is another family just waiting and wondering.

Problems as the child gets older

For older children the more noticeable difficulties often centre on planning or perception problems. One of the most difficult things for children, and parents, to deal with is the inability to think and plan ahead. Coupled with hardship in reading, writing and speech this means that as a child gets older the hidden handicap is more evident. This is why it is such an advantage if the child has earlier been in an environment where the struggles have been noticed and handled in such a way that he does not already have a feeling of being 'odd' or 'peculiar'. I mentioned how Daniel at four years old has already drawn back from trying new or difficult activities. We also saw how right Anna was to find the most helpful nursery for Daniel. If, instead, she had glossed over the difficulties of this little boy she would have left him open to harsher treatment later. Perhaps in an environment where he may have come up against those who had no time for a child with difficulties in climbing, tying shoelaces and PE.

Sophie took her 3-year-old to the doctor because she kept falling over, but an appointment with an orthopaedic man showed nothing. So 'nothing' was done for the next two years. Meanwhile Sophie became more and more concerned about Hanna, especially as she was slow to develop speech. However, Sophie said that as Hanna seemed to understand very well what was said to her, and as everyone else was saying, 'Don't worry, don't fuss,' Sophie tried not to get het up. 'I truly regret not making a big fuss much earlier,' she said. Once Hanna started primary school and was expected to sit down when told, to tie her own shoelaces and to 'keep up', then the trouble started.

Help may be sought and offered by a variety of professions – an educational psychologist, a physiotherapist, an occupational therapist or a speech and language therapist. 'We have tried them all, and the professionals we have consulted seem so vague,' said Richard. 'Nothing seems to make much difference. Perhaps Bob is just clumsy, and there it is. He just seems disconnected in some way.' Richard had been called to the school when Bob's teacher had become worried as she believed Bob has specific learning difficulties. Richard had also spoken to another parent and compared notes. Richard's concern was that the other child with several similar symptoms had been diagnosed as autistic, but Richard held on to the belief that his little boy loved contact and communication and therefore was not part of the autistic spectrum.

What you should do

For a pre-school child the first person to talk to should be your GP or health visitor, and a request should be made for a referral to a paediatrician or a child development centre. An assessment can then be made by a psychologist, physiotherapist, speech and language therapist or an occupational therapist. Once your child begins nursery or school it is advisable to seek their help and explain to them the tasks your child finds most difficult. You may even need to print out information about this condition and give copies to the school.

Unfortunately help is often limited because of scarce resources, so parents told me how they had found ways of providing support themselves: 'Plenty of ball games', 'Rough and tumble', 'Swimming lessons', 'Play-doh and finger painting', 'Speech therapy, if you can afford it, is a must', 'Keep in with the SENCO (special educational needs co-ordinator)' and 'Talk to other parents and explain what dyspraxia is'.

The most important thing, though, seems to be that children should be helped to remain confident so that their self-esteem does not suffer. Watch out for signs of frustration in your child when he finds he is unable to do all the things he wants to do. If you and your child are prepared to find as many strategies as you can to develop co-ordination, organizational skills and other difficulties, the problems will not accumulate. The co-operation of the school is essential. Also, new technological advances can be wonderful. Indeed, children with many different special needs find that a computer has become a godsend in helping them overcome motor difficulties.

The prognosis is usually hopeful, because although dyspraxia is not curable, increased maturity means there will be improvement in some areas. I heard from many parents who told me that their children did overcome many of their early difficulties.

Helping a child with dyspraxia
- Don't accept the label of an 'over-fussy mother' if you believe there is a problem for your child.
- Become a 'voice' by explaining to as many people as you can what dyspraxia is and how it affects a child.
- By raising awareness of this condition you will create a better general understanding of the resources needed by dyspraxic children.
- Remember life may be hard for your child, so watch out for him being tired and frustrated by tasks he cannot complete.
- Physical games, rough and tumble, and sports like swimming are found to be particularly helpful.

12

Dyslexia

I am all I think
Thoughts –
Like bees buzzing around my head
I am all these things
I am like a person trapped in a maze
And these are my walls
But one day I will find my way out
And I'll be free . . .

(Georgina Ellis, aged 12,
who has overcome dyslexia)

The meaning of dyslexia

The word 'dyslexia' comes from the Greek and means 'difficulty with words'. According to the British Dyslexia Association one in ten children suffer from this invisible handicap but more than 70 per cent of schools have no teachers qualified to teach dyslexic pupils. The BDA is the voice of dyslexic people, and their national helpline (www.bda-dyslexia.org.uk) handles more than 40,000 enquiries a year.

Early signs to look for are:

- putting clothes on the wrong way round
- difficulty learning nursery rhymes
- difficulty in learning the alphabet
- getting words muddled
- forgetting the names of friends or teachers
- pleasure in listening to stories but showing no desire to learn to read
- difficulty in sticking things together, threading beads and making things
- poor sense of direction
- poor auditory memory sequencing.

Of all the hidden disabilities I discuss in this book, dyslexia is the most widely acknowledged and known about. Considering that it usually affects reading ability in one way or another, it is surprising how so many people in the artistic and even literary worlds are prepared to consider themselves dyslexic! Some people with dyslexia cannot learn to read at all. The rest have problems, from mild to very severe, with reading, spelling and reversal of symbols. A great many dyslexic children get a confused picture of the print on a page, and it is believed that the difficulties can be either phonological or visual or a mixture of the two. The first indication of dyslexia for you as a parent may well be that your child enjoys being read to, but shows no interest in letters or words. Or you may notice that he has difficulty learning nursery rhymes (although this *may* be an indication of difficulty with short-term memory). A more serious sign is if your child has some difficulties in development of speech and language, but this could be due to a motor problem. It is only when a cluster of *different* difficulties appear that you should begin to consider the possibility of dyslexia.

Let me repeat once again: children develop skills at very different rates of accomplishment, and your child may only need a little extra help and time when learning the letters of the alphabet. Don't be too alarmed if one of your children is a little slower in learning to read than the others were – like all the milestones connected with childhood, there is a great variance in when the ability to understand letters comes about. From my own experience as a mother I remember that one of my children seemed to 'know' how to read almost from one day to the next. When my next child began to struggle over letters I recall being puzzled about why she had to use so much effort. But, all that she needed was a bit more time than her brother, and within six months was well on the way to reading. So don't be too hasty to make the diagnosis of a 'problem'. I should have known better than to use one child's achievement as a bench mark for another!

Making an early start

The Government in the UK has acknowledged the scale of the problem and has announced that they are 'committed to effecting a culture change in schools to overturn years of neglect towards children with this condition'. Once again, however, provision of help at the present time is very patchy according to where you live. The government guidelines which sound so positive also depend upon the interpretation which a local education authority puts on its policy. Many parents feel very let down, as 'appropriate help' seems to mean different things in different areas.

The ruling in the House of Lords (31 July 2000) puts increased pressure on schools to take dyslexia seriously. This ruling has enormous implications for teachers and psychologists in that it *'insists they have a personal duty to care for their pupils and not simply a responsibility to answer or to advise the local education authority'* [my italics]. A duty of care means that teachers, and psychologists, can be held accountable for their advice and actions, such as failing to recognize a pupil's dyslexia. The Dyslexia Institute believes that justice is available now, retrospectively, for all those for whom no help was on offer earlier.

Dyslexia, which is a most common invisible disability, seems to cause heartache to many parents and children. For parents, because until their child begins to learn to read they may have no idea that there is a problem at all. While for children it is hard when they fail to master one more skill which their peers manage to take in their stride.

A special needs teacher who contributed her expertise and understanding to this book when discussing dyslexia repeated what has been said so often about other hidden disabilities: it is important for a child to get help *before* there are any psychological issues arising from a sense of failure.

As we have heard from Andrea, she was bewildered when her third child seemed unwilling (or unable?) to grasp the concept of reading. Dyslexia to varying degrees often seems to run in families, and it is now believed that a gene may be responsible for this.

As always an early diagnosis can help and it is beneficial for you as a parent to consult a professional who will help you understand the *way* your child learns (but beware of a fixed label of dyslexia at too early an age). 'I feel dreadful about the way I dealt with Marie in those early days. I couldn't believe she couldn't remember her letters and I know I shouted at her. I just thought she was being silly.' Rachel said this to me, and I know many parents reading this will have 'been there' too.

You may find your child muddles left from right, finds it hard to copy from the board, and has a poor visual or auditory memory of varying degrees. All this can be very hard for a parent to deal with, especially, as I have commented earlier, if up until now your child has passed through all the previous developmental phases with ease.

Looking back to their own childhoods there are parents who recall they were slower than their peers to read fluently. Jake was one father who talked with me. He remembers that he found reading a mystery and almost gave up on the whole thing. Luckily he had an uncle who took him to one side and said that reading was important and would open the gates to many wonderful and exciting things. This intrigued Jake and he spent hours and hours forcing himself to understand letters and, in time, to read. He said it makes him wonder what would have happened if he had not learnt every trick available to aid his reading. I wondered if 'uncle' had had some problems too, and knew what it was like for an adult to be handi-capped in this way. When Jake in turn could see that his child had some problems with reading he was on to it right away and looked for advice. The help Jake found for his son meant patching the left eye; in this way a child with unstable binocular control can improve eye control and find reading much easier.

Patrick was hit at school each time he stumbled over a word and he had dreadful memories of how he became the butt of jokes from teachers and children. The humiliation he felt over forty years ago has left scars which are still all too visible, but as a father he channelled his anger into finding early appropriate help for his two children. He said that although he now realizes that non-invasive scans and an understanding of genes show there are some physical reasons for dyslexia, he still burns with shame at how as a lad in Ireland his poor reading skills were equated with him 'being stupid'.

Polly told me that because her daughter has *mild* dyslexia the fact that there was a problem at all was not appreciated until at the age of eight Maxine said that the letters on the blackboard kept jumping about. On investigation at an eye hospital Polly was told her daughter had 'brain fatigue'. In fact it meant that Maxine was struggling to make sense of what she was seeing, and eventually an educational psychologist diagnosed mild dyslexia. This mother told me that a *mild form of dyslexia*, compared to all invisible disabilities of differing severity, means that you will really have to struggle to get extra help. Even after the diagnosis had been made, and the school informed her that Maxine suffered from a bad short-term memory, this child still received detentions for forgetting things. 'I have been up to the school, and wept in front of the head, about the way they treat her. But because it is a *mild* disorder it keeps being "forgotten about" or because there is nothing to see when you look at my daughter people don't believe there is anything wrong.'

Angie agreed that finding help for a child with mild dyslexia is a problem. 'Nobody will take you, or your child, seriously. I know that a kind and patient teacher can encourage my daughter – I have seen the results and I know she is bright. Put her in a class where the teacher has a different style and her brain freezes.'

Again, I heard from parents who said they swung from believing 'nothing is wrong with my child' to *knowing* that something was up'. Caroline: 'Oh, I now call a spade a spade and say I knew something was wrong with my child.' But somehow it is not easy for parents to acknowledge that there is a problem connected with reading; it immediately engenders a feeling of 'shame' – a word I heard many times from parents. So, be on the lookout to make sure your child does not begin to feel this too; many parents reported to me that this can be the beginning of your child's self-esteem plummeting to zero.

You will hear from other parents about children who were late-starters; what this usually implies is that the child managed to learn some special strategies along the way to cope with his difficulties. Especially so if a child was unsure whether to use his left or right hand for writing, games and other activities. There are too many stories from adults who suffered (and I do mean suffered) from dyslexia when growing up. This nearly always went unrecognized so they were considered to have learning difficulties. 'I knew I was clever, yet I got put in with the dumbos.' 'I worked so hard, but was always marked down for spelling and handwriting.' 'Stumbling over reading cast a blight over my life.' 'I gave up writing essays because they always came back covered in red crosses because of the spelling.' These are only a few of the many comments like this made to me by adults.

Barney told me that, as an adult, he has daily problems with not being able to read accurately and of the accompanying embarrass-ment he still feels. His many stories of his experiences as a child and adolescent make one's flesh crawl. Somehow the inability to read fluently goes hand in hand with 'dull', and Barney knows only too well how this shattered his self-confidence. It was only when his little boy showed signs which Barney recognized all too clearly that he began to think that perhaps it was not too late for him to get help too. It takes a lot of pluck to go back into the education system where previous experiences have been marred by failure. But, he believed he was in a unique position to help his son, and together they are looking for strategies and support. 'First of all,' said Barney, 'you have to know and accept that you are dyslexic.' He told me that he would have given a great deal to have been told this as a child. He also remembered how by trying to hide the fact that he was struggling he became anxious, and that made the problem worse.

Helping children to cope

A teacher who works exclusively with children with these problems told me that as a child she had to cope alone with her own dyslexia. She worked out an explanation for herself which was that 'the wires were crossed in my head'. When one day she read an article about dyslexia, she was overjoyed to recognize the signs and to say, 'That's what I've got!' She learnt some strategies, such as wearing a ring on one finger to remind her to use the correct hand. Mrs W says her pupils are thrilled to know that she, too, is dyslexic and *really* understands what it is like not to know whether to turn left or right, which hand to use for table tennis, and to forget things others expect her to remember! She urges parents to seek help to discover whether a child is an auditory or visual learner, since this will enable him to find the best way of going forward. Mrs W also said that she still finds it hard to drive across town or to find her car in the car park.

As with most disabilities, there are swings and roundabouts concerning help on offer. One parent said that as nobody dies from dyslexia there is often no money available for the help that these children need.

Once again, the issue is whether or not the outside world is sympathetic and understanding about this invisible handicap. 'No, No, No,' said the majority of parents, 'they are not.' 'And neither are the schools,' went on the chorus. 'It beats me,' said Mike, 'it seems as if the school sees it as a reflection upon themselves to say a child is dyslexic.'

Gladys told me, with incredulity, that the day she received an official letter from the school saying that they could see no evidence of her child being dyslexic, a school report arrived which said her daughter 'had difficulties keeping up, didn't concentrate, and constantly forgot things'.

When Ruth talked to me about her daughter, who is now sixteen, she told me of a catalogue of difficulties. She was another who believed that because Paula has *mild* dyslexia she was denied the help she needed. At nursery and primary school nothing was picked up, except to report that Paula was careless. The knock-on effect of this was that Paula was often reluctant to have a go at things, and the more trouble that Paula got into at school, the more stressed she became and the worse the symptoms were. Eventually Ruth managed to get the special needs teacher to see Paula, but the report was that 'there were no signs of dyslexia', and meanwhile Paula became more and more unhappy at school. She found it harder to concentrate when under stress, which resulted in more detentions. 'We were caught in a vicious circle,' said Ruth. Because the report had been unhelpful for Paula, she was denied extra time in examinations. Ruth could see 'failure' on the cards. 'Do you know that 50 per cent of young offenders are dyslexic?' she continued. 'No wonder, when they were probably made to feel stupid and careless at school.'

Once again, this parent had to turn to the private sector for help and an educational psychologist diagnosed Paula as dyslexic. 'Phew,' said Ruth, 'once you have got a bit of paper, you're in, so please, please tell any other parent to go for a proper diagnosis. Just think of the stress that Paula was under all those years.' Ruth told me that dyslexia had been explained to her in this way: 'Say a boat had a hole in it, you might be able to keep it afloat in the water, but burden it and it sinks. That's Paula all over.' She said she could cry remembering that Paula had been told in class to 'pull your socks up' time and time again. 'Question, question and question again,' said Ruth. 'And don't wait until your child is in secondary school; they won't be interested then as there is no funding for help.'

As we heard from Amy, her son was only diagnosed with dyslexia when he reached university, and more than once I heard of children struggling until someone at their college or place of further education asked why this problem had not been picked up earlier.

You may also be thrown by your child asking you, '*Why* can't I read?' And you may have difficulties in knowing how to help. It is vitally important for the mental health of a child who is struggling in this way to be told that even though there may be major problems with reading, writing, spelling or maths he or she is not careless or stupid. The child may take some convincing, so it is paramount that *you* believe this. There is a great deal to be said for looking at the positive side too: children who are dyslexic often show a high degree of creativity and a surprisingly large number of our most gifted artists and designers are also dyslexic.

Although dyslexia cannot be cured, there are many ways that a child can be helped which will allow other abilities to be recognized. This is why it is so important for this 'invisible' handicap to be understood early on in a child's life. Learning in different ways should be encouraged, and, as I have already said, it is extremely important that an early sense of failure does not permeate every area of learning.

Audrey told us in an earlier chapter how frantic she became when Liam couldn't remember words like 'the', 'that', 'can' and 'would', and if this is a problem you and your child are facing you may find a book called *The Gift of Dyslexia* a very worthwhile read, although several people who are dyslexic told me they found the title irritating because they do not take well to being told they have a gift. However, the author Ronald Davis – who is himself dyslexic – puts a positive spin on dyslexia because he believes that it is beneficial for all people with dyslexia to know that their minds work in exactly the same way as many people who were geniuses. He believes that people with dyslexia are highly aware of their environment and are more curious than average, and that they think mainly in pictures rather than words. Of course, in his book he also looks at the negative side, at the link between a dyslexic child who is curious and inquisitive and who will only give his attention to what most interests him. If a child is not engaged in his school work, he may be bored and either daydream or become distracted and even hyperactive, reactions which could lead to a diagnosis of ADD or ADHD.

The Gift of Dyslexia has lists of words which many children who are dyslexic have difficulty with and the parents who recommended this book said they found knowing about these 'trigger words' most helpful. The author gives a clear and understandable explanation just why there are words which cause some children particular problems.

I spoke to Rose, a young girl of fourteen, knowing that she had struggled with reading and spelling difficulties for several years. I showed her the list of trigger words which she recognized immediately. Although now she reads fluently she can remember in the past skipping over these words, and then wondering why a page had not made sense. Rose has been fortunate enough to be at a school which recognizes that early intervention and help is vital and one-to-one tuition has been there for Rose from the age of five. I asked her if seeing a special needs teacher during the school day had caused her any problems at school. She laughed at me and said, 'No, why should it? I just need a bit of extra help, that's all.'

If only more schools had this attitude and support available. Polly, whose daughter has ME and who is also dyslexic, understood the Government's guidelines to mean that if a child was absent from school due to illness for more than fifteen working days then educational help should be available 'sooner rather than later'. The school will need to ask the parents to provide a doctor's note or a consultant's letter and seek support for the referral from the school's medical officer confirming ill health. She also understood the guidelines to mean her child would receive a minimum of five hours home tuition. However, on investigation, she was informed it would be five hours maximum. The fact that her daughter is also dyslexic did not mean that there would be additional help. Polly was geared up for one more fight but felt thwarted by red tape when all she heard was, 'We are sympathetic but . . .' and 'We would like to offer more but . . .'.

As with dyspraxia, a child who is dyslexic and feels disorientated may appear clumsy. Although this will manifest itself over a wide range of levels, be on the look out if your child shows awkward or ungainly behaviour. A child may also find it difficult to know his way around very familiar places and easily get lost. Rose told me that when she was four she was taken to a theme park where children were allowed to 'drive' a car around a toy city. All the other children managed the roundabouts and the road layouts. Rose did not. At the time her family and the other children laughed at the way she was the only one going the wrong way. She remembers that she had no idea what to do, and couldn't understand how the other children knew how to 'drive' around the town safely. Sad to hear that ten years on she remembers the laughter. I am sorry to say that, as her grandmother, I was one of the adults who thought it was all in a day's fun, and had no idea we were watching a child with a serious difficulty in knowing which way to turn.

Parents can become bemused and hopeful by media reports such as 'Is Dyslexia Beaten?' In this article in the *Mail on Sunday*, exercises designed for astronauts who suffer from temporary dyslexia in space are alleged to help improve the co-ordination of children. Further research is now under way, but while media attention is to be welcomed, and such a headline can lift the hearts of many parents, it can also add pressure on already worried parents wondering if there is yet one more avenue they should explore. It is confusing when an already tried programme is heralded as 'new' and 'phenomenal'.

Scientists are now developing a new way to help diagnose dyslexia: by measuring whether children's eyes work properly when they read. The kit measures 'eye wobble', one of the key components of dyslexia. A computer link shows whether the child's eyes are steady or whether they wobble. This discovery will make it possible to gauge if a child can fix his eyes for the fleeting second which is needed to read words. John Stein, a professor of neurology, believes that more than half of the children who are dyslexic have eye-control problems. Exercises, patching one eye (if eyes are competing to take the lead) and even wearing coloured glasses may all help. These treatments must, it goes without saying, be carried out under medical supervision.

There are simple tests, too, which can give teachers and parents early warning: difficulties with bead-threading, spotting words which rhyme, and remembering numbers can all help with an early diagnosis. Sadly the BDA says their evidence is that too many children are not diagnosed until they fail to learn to read, and thus precious time is lost. Use of the spell-check on a computer has become a wonderful aid to any person who has dyslexic features, and schools are aware of this.

No longer is dyslexia called as it once was the 'middle-class disease' since there is now proof that there are physical causes.

Some facts about dyslexia
- Seventy per cent of those affected are male.
- Remember that 4 per cent of the population is severely dyslexic.
- A further 6 per cent have mild to moderate problems.
- Dyslexia occurs in people from all backgrounds and abilities.
- Dyslexic people may also have problems with co-ordination and short-term memory.
- Be alert to the fact that poor self-image and low self-esteem will cause additional problems.
- There is a strong overlap between dyslexia and dyspraxia.

13

Special educational needs

He has a deal of learning but it never lies straight.
(Dr Samuel Johnson)

Learning difficulties or learning differences?

The term 'Special Educational Needs' was introduced in the UK in the 1981 Education Act, and the DfES (Department for Education and Skills) estimate that around one in five children nationally have a special educational need at some point in their school career. If the need cannot be met by the school, the child is entitled to additional support. So, you should keep abreast of different legislative changes and a good way to do this is to access the DfES SEN pages on the excellent website (www.dfee.gov.uk). Familiarize yourself with the code of practice and the difference between the five-stage model for SEN assessment and provision. Also be sure you understand the term Individual Education Plan (IEP). You should be aware that the direction nowadays is to include all children together in a mainstream school, with additional help for some children. This is being reinforced by legislation in the UK. Another first-class website to provide you with more information and to spell out the different steps you can take is Tiger Child (www.tiger child.com).

The term you will have heard is 'LD'. So what *is* LD? Is it 'learning disorder', 'learning difficulties', 'learning disabled' or learning differences'? I prefer the newer term 'learning differences' because it moves away from the negative aspect of the problem. There are different types of LD, the range is from mild to profound, so you may be confronted by SLD (severe learning difficulties) or MLD (mild learning difficulties). The most important factor with any learning difficulty is that it should be picked up as early as possible so that appropriate help can be given. Learning difficulties occur in children of all backgrounds and abilities, and more boys than girls are diagnosed with LD.

These are the signs which may point to a child having learning difficulties:

- language: talking later than peers and with pronunciation problems
- failure to make a start in school subjects
- difficulty in concentrating and being easily distracted
- poor handwriting
- poor social skills
- slow to learn new skills
- poor co-ordination or perceptual motor disability.

Of course, many parents may have noticed that their child has some of these difficulties – but once again it is only when there is a cluster of such difficulties that a parent should begin to wonder about LD. It is often in the area of learning difficulties that parents who *are* worried and ask for help early on are told, 'There is nothing to worry about.' And in many cases this is true and they do find that their children catch up with their peers. On the other hand children with mild LD may never be diagnosed as having a problem, and may have to struggle throughout their time at school. Non-diagnosis of mild LD may account for the number of secondary school children who drop out of education. Early diagnosis and intervention helps a child to cope more easily, by developing different skills and strategies.

The children who are identified as having LD are often the children who have problems learning at school, but may well shine in other areas. Unfortunately for them, though, there is a tremendous focus on academic ability today and many such children suffer on account of this. As there is a wide variation in the range of LD, you may find that your child has amazing pockets of ability, especially in creative areas.

Joey: 'My daughter has a low IQ. We got help when she was little but now nobody wants to know. Luckily we have got together with other parents and that has empowered us.'

Caroline: 'My daughter has a rare genetic disorder. When I asked about her learning difficulties I was told that in a working-class family she would not be out of place. I was appalled.'

Thomas: 'Muddle, MUDDLE, MUDDLE until we paid for a private appointment. Her speech was delayed and so was her walking. We are waiting now for her to be statemented.'

Louisa: 'It's not *now* that worries us. We can cope. It is the future.'

LD children are not 'stupid'

There is still much misunderstanding about LD and even today there are people who class all LD children as 'stupid'. As I mentioned in the chapter on gifted children (chapter 9) it is possible to have LD and at the same time be highly gifted in other ways. Children with LD process information differently but this does not prevent them very often being of average or even above average intelligence. A child with LD may perform poorly for a number of reasons in the standard tests which most children take; so it is important not to rely solely on the assessments from these.

'All people have learning curves, all students with disABILITIES have strengths and talents that are often overlooked by their learning obstacles . . . there must be a balance of the two,' says Barbara Day. Take a look at her excellent website, Guide to Special Education (www.SpecialEd.About.com), where teachers, parents and students may find answers to help them overcome obstacles and move on to success.

While the move is now towards all children being taught in mainstream schools, children with severe mental and physical disabilities may need to be placed in a special school or unit. Special Educational Provision is for a child who finds it harder to learn than other children. If your child is in a mainstream school watch out for teasing or bullying from other pupils; and make sure that any extra help provided is appropriate and really aids your child.

Network 81 (www.network81.co.uk) is a national network of parents working towards properly resourced inclusive education for children with special needs. Look at their website or telephone their helpline (0870 770 3306) for more information. There is an annual membership fee of £15 but worth supporting if you agree with their aim: to advance the education of children with special needs, and to educate parents of such children about all matters relating to the education of their children.

Maggie: 'My boy was entitled to a classroom assistant but it seemed to me that they spent most of the school day excluded from the class and just wandering around. So watch out.'

Clara: 'My child qualified for a one-to-one helper, but it was a dinner-lady, not someone who knew about special needs.'

Harold: ' I found that as the kids got older they were less sympathetic to my child and the problems increased. Anyone with a speech impediment seems set up for being made a butt of jokes. And *why* do people think that speech problems and being "dim" always go hand in hand?' Harold also believed that it is not only kids who equate LD with being 'dumb' or 'retarded'.

'Of *course* I get upset from time to time when I see she struggles with things. But we have decided that it is up to us to make sure she feels comfortable with herself and is never made to feel she is not up to the mark.'

Parents told me how important it is to talk with their child about the things which they find particularly difficult, and to give some explanation of why this is so. Above all, listen to your child; you may be horrified to discover that he feels different and worries about how to fit in. Other concerns may spring from believing that nobody understands; and by talking together this will help to dispel this anxiety. Marianna Csoti's book *Social Awareness Skills for Children* will be useful for any parent who wants to help their child improve his social understanding and awareness, and to give a boost to his self-esteem.

So, explain as much as you can and don't treat your child's LD as a family secret; make sure every family member knows the areas where your child needs extra help. Unfortunately, you won't be able to protect your child all the time from the outside world, which can be very uncaring and cruel, but you can help him to develop as many coping skills as possible.

If your child's difficulties are in the social skills he may on occasion act inappropriately, perhaps by being 'too friendly'. As a parent you should step in and give a clear explanation to your child of why this behaviour doesn't go down too well. You may also need to give clear guidelines about how to make – and keep – friends. Explain that it is harder for some than it is for others to do this.

If you are concerned that your child has a speech, language or communication difficulty contact the Afasic helpline (08453 55 55 77) or www.afasic.org.uk, where you will find a wealth of information about speech and language therapy. There are helpful explanations about the different areas of language learning and different forms of language impairment. Some children have difficulty in understanding language, some in using language, and some in both understanding *and* using language. Visit the website LD Information at www.ldinfo.com – plenty of good material there.

Through help and support on all sides many learning differences can be overcome, so an alliance between parents and teachers is vital. And don't forget to keep in touch with your health visitor, often a good source of local help and resources.

Lastly, it's as well to remember that we all find learning and doing *some* things easier than others.

Dos and don'ts for coping with learning differences

- Remember there are different types of learning difficulties which range from mild to profound.
- Early diagnosis of even mild LD is important.
- Don't overprotect – you will not be doing your child a favour.
- Don't put too much faith in academic tests.
- Don't let up on discipline.
- Don't make the mistake of thinking only *you* understand how your child is feeling.
- Do be assertive on your child's behalf.
- Be realistic about your child's strengths and weaknesses.
- Encourage your child's 'strengths' to compensate for weaker processing skills.
- *Talk* to your child about areas which are difficult for him and try to explain *why*.
- *Listen* and try to understand the worries your child has about their LD.
- Provide guidelines for making friends, and keeping them.
- Make it clear to your child what behaviour is acceptable and what is not.
- Find out about any resources and help you are entitled to.
- Don't treat your child's difficulties as a family secret.
- Talk to the SENCO (special educational needs co-ordinator) or school nurse at your child's school.

Home schooling

Although education in the UK is compulsory, school is not, and more parents are now considering home schooling for their children. For some it is because they are not happy with the education on offer, especially if their child has a special need. In other circumstances, rightly or wrongly, other parents are convinced it is the best way to proceed.

'We educate because we like the lifestyle. We can be spontaneous and respond to the needs and moods of our children. It is pure freedom,' says Melissa Hill, author of bestselling *Smart Woman's Guide to Staying at Home*. 'We treat the world as our classroom.'

'Teachers are asked to do too much,' said Roger. 'They are expected to act as nurses, watch out for each child with a range of "special needs", keep up to the mark, oh, and teach them too. We decided that as a family we were in a better place to teach, and support, our boys who have ADHD.' Of course, Roger is right when he says that the shortage of school nurses is forcing teachers, who are not always willing, to administer treatments to children with medical problems.

'Emily was awarded extra support but the job of a special needs assistant is so poorly paid and has so little respect or value, it was no help whatsoever. We had to take Emily out of school and have never regretted it. No more fights with the authorities.'

'I woke up one morning and wondered why I was spending all my time clashing with authorities to "provide" for my daughter when we could do it better ourselves. We have never looked back.'

'No longer will he be in detention all day. No longer will he be called dummy and worse. No longer will he be teased for the weight gain caused by his medication. No more will he be harassed and tripped in the hallway. No more defeating report cards. We will take our time and there will be no pressure. Yippee!'

Pinky McKay who wrote *Parenting by Heart* is very much in favour of home schooling. 'My son was diagnosed as both "gifted" *and* "learning disabled" by a school psychologist at the age of six. He was put in the lowest group where he saw himself as a slow learner and developed an "I can't do this" attitude. Later when I deschooled him at age eleven, he was barely reading and was convinced he was "dumb". Within six weeks he was following the stocks and shares in the newspaper. I believe home schooling is the best thing for a child who marches to a different drum, because his talents lay outside of what was normally valued within the schooling system. He is very artistic and now has a degree in interior design.' Pinky McKay has her own website (www.pinky-mychild.com)

which anyone wanting to know more on this subject will find interesting.

If home schooling is something you are considering you should contact the Home Education Advisory Service (www.heas.org.uk). Members of the charity HEAS have access to an advice line for curriculum guidance, and a specialist Dyslexia Helpline. The DfES sets out conditions parents have to fulfil in order to educate their child at home; these can be seen on their website (www.dfes.gov.uk). The Scottish Charity Schoolhouse Association, established in 1996, has a 24-hour information line on 0870 745 0967 and will be helpful to any parent involved in home schooling; visit their website (www.schoolhouse.org.uk). In the US there is www.homeschool yellowpages.com/NFHEE/webrings.html for up-to-the-minute advice.

If you want to have a glimpse of the future in education look at www.dfes.gov/uk/ictfutures, where the school of the future will be an ICT-rich environment. One of the considerations is whether there will be 'opportunities for learners with special needs to participate fully, for example through developments in voice-activated software and touch sensitive screen technologies'. Fine! Particularly if 'transforming the way we learn' also takes into account that every child learns in his own special way.

Toilet training

This is a particular aspect of learning difficulties which requires special attention. Most parents are prepared for the cleaning up and training of a toddler – all part of bringing up baby. It is harder when the child passes the toddler stage and yet is not dry or clean. Children who have poor communication skills and limited control over their bodies will find it hardest of all. So toilet training can very often become a difficult problem for children with disabilities.

As with younger children, it is important to be in tune with the child so that signs may be picked up about whether he needs the potty or lavatory. Try to pace yourself to your child's timing, which may not be the one you would have chosen. Keep in mind that it may only be extra time that your child needs to master this skill.

You will probably have already read with your child one of the several story books which show by example how a child should be potty trained. You should make sure your child knows the words the family use for the toilet and the different functions, and if your child is cared for by a sitter or another member of the family make them familiar with the words or signs your child may use.

Powerful social pressures exist about cleanliness and if your child – past the toddler stage – has a problem then it is important to get all the help you can. It is as well to get some professional advice sooner rather than later, to ensure there are no medical problems which are at the root of the incontinence. Although children with a physical disability may be embarrassed by their incontinence, I heard from other parents whose concern is for their children who do not seem to notice, or care too much, if they wet or soil.

A mother who has a daughter with a severe degree of learning difficulty told me that although at three years old her daughter did indicate when she was wet, now at nine she doesn't seem to notice. It is often when a child is six or seven or older and still not out of nappies that both mother and child can begin to feel isolated by this. There are fewer invitations to other children's homes, and even babysitters begin to be less than willing to help. 'It's the not talking about it which is so dreadful,' said Sue. 'All my family know that Trev has a problem, probably Asperger's, but they only ever talk about his odd way of talking, never anything about what else we have to deal with. At seven he is still in nappies.' So parents have to deal with a kind of taboo about what is spoken about, and what is not.

From others I heard of children who are sufficiently aware to hide or conceal in some way the fact that they have wet or soiled themselves. However, they will not indicate in advance that they need to use a lavatory. Claudia told me that her daughter, who is at the severe end of the autistic spectrum, could signal to them when her bladder was full, but any bowel movement frightened her – she hated the feeling of something leaving her body.

A study was carried out by Judith Cavet for the Joseph Rowntree Foundation called *People Don't Understand: Children, Young People and Their Families Living with a Hidden Disability*. The hidden disability she describes is around the experiences of families whose children are affected by faecal incontinence as a result of physical impairment. Although her study was with families of children who suffered from syndromes such as spina bifida or Hirschsprung's disease, much of the ground she covers applies just as well to families with a child with less obvious disabilities. Cavet quotes from parents she interviewed who, like many parents of a child with special needs, have children or a young person generally seen as non-disabled and often treated as such. The lack of an easily recognizable disability had many of the implications I have already discussed.

Lizzie said that at times she almost longs for her child to show some outward sign of a disability, because with an invisible one there is no sympathy for an older child who appears to have had an 'accident'. Lizzie told me that only the week before she had had to rush her child into a lavatory and used the one marked 'disabled'. When they came out they were met with the fury of a woman who scolded them for using the facilities. How was she to reply? Lizzie wanted to shout, 'My son *is* disabled,' but thought it may upset Edward. Once more we see the daily issues which can and do arise. It is as well to be prepared for incidents like this.

One of the most difficult areas for Brenda to deal with was when her daughter became fascinated and absorbed with faeces. Every bowel movement brought about a fight between mother and child as Emily wanted to smear around and hold every stool. 'That is when it became clear to me that only I could really care for Emily. No one else would.' This kind of behaviour is an even more hidden side of caring for a child with special needs. And a side which is rarely spoken about. Until this time Brenda had found her friends and family very supportive, but Emily's new preoccupation was considered to be beyond the scope of babysitters and grandparents.

The mainstream school which Maddie attended coped quite well with her educationally, but the physical care which she needed at times meant that she was reassessed and moved to a school for children with special needs. 'Not that that was ever given as the reason,' said her mother. This has had a disastrous outcome for Maddie because having learnt to read simple books in the mainstream school, she is now given only picture books and seems to be losing her capacity to read.

Parents who have been faced by this problem advise you to check out to see if your local authority will provide free help with nappies or incontinence pads – many will once a child is past three years old.

Hints for parents about toilet training
- Make sure there is no physical reason for incontinence.
- Remember your child may just need more time to cope with bodily functions.
- Discuss the situation with the nursery or school.
- Don't be embarrassed to ask for help.
- Find out if there is any practical help on offer in your area.

14

Depression

In disease medical men guess: if they cannot ascertain a disease they call it nervous.

(John Keats)

Children get depressed too

Depression in children is perhaps the most obviously overlooked invisible disability. There are adults who do not believe that children can get depressed, and think that depression is a 'grown-up thing'.

There are many different reasons for depression – both for children and adults; one incident alone or a cluster of factors can trigger off feelings of hopelessness or despair. Stress and depression often go hand in hand, so it would be foolish not to realize that children are affected by the knock-on effect when their parents are trying to cope with their own stress. Unfortunately, there are many parents who won't let themselves think that their child is depressed, so it very often goes untreated. For example, when a family breakup happens there are mothers and fathers who so want to believe that their children will not be affected, that they cling to the hope that 'children adjust' and 'don't notice'. Sadly, they *do* notice, and often have to suffer in silence.

Possible causes of depression in a child include:

- losing a parent or grandparent
- death of a pet
- being bullied
- having a stressed or depressed parent
- moving house
- birth of a new baby in the family
- breakup of a family
- being abused sexually, physically or emotionally
- dealing with learning or developmental difficulties
- being physically ill
- convalescing in a weak state after an illness
- concern about performance at school
- difficulties with exams and tests
- failure to make relationships and have friends
- worrying about the future.

Of course, very young children cannot tell us how they feel, but they *show* us by their behaviour. So a small child may suddenly become clinging, develop eating problems and have disturbed sleep. They may have nightmares or tantrums, and regress to wetting or soiling themselves. School-age children may find it hard to concentrate, develop sleep problems, become 'difficult' at home or at school, and even stop playing or wanting to go to school. A mysterious 'tummy ache' which comes and goes may well be a sign of your child's distress and inner turmoil.

Older children may show signs of being moody and uncooperative. But adolescents often are like this anyway, so how can you tell? Look for additional signs such as giving up all outside interests, not keeping up with friends, eating problems, or acting recklessly. Keep a look-out, too, for negative thoughts about the future. Irritability can be mistaken for rudeness. Recently there has been an increase in the number of teenage suicides – the number has more than doubled in the past twenty years.

According to the Mental Health Foundation 2 per cent of children under the age of twelve have some form of depression, compared with 5 per cent of teenagers. As many as 8 to 11 per cent of children and young people experience anxiety to such an extent that it affects their ability to get on with their everyday lives. It is calculated that at any one time 20 per cent of children experience psychological problems.

Parents of children who have Asperger syndrome, unrecognized dyslexia, ME or other invisible problems firmly believe that depression comes *because* of these disabilities, exacerbated by the reaction of the adults around them. In these cases, depression is actually an expedient reaction to a situation and if the signs are read correctly will prompt a cry for help. If you know your child as well as you should, and if you are on the look-out, you will recognize the difference between ordinary unhappiness and a serious bout of depression. Keep an eye out, too, for a child who suddenly becomes unaccountably disruptive; bad behaviour is often a tell-tale sign of underlying depression.

Ways of finding help

Fiona: 'My daughter had a great deal of trouble at school – as we found out later because her learning problems were not recognized. When she became depressed I went to our GP. She agreed with me that medication was not appropriate and was undecided at first about where to refer her. Eventually Sylvia saw the practice counsellor. That helped. But they could only provide six sessions. Once the counselling stopped she was not so well, but the school said that as she was finished with the counsellor they must have thought she was no longer depressed and so she should return to school.'

Judy: 'I ignored the signs. I didn't want to think a child of mine could get depressed. How I regret waiting to look for help. Once I did, there was a long waiting list for a NHS referral to a child psychotherapist. We had to go privately.'

Yet James, aged thirteen, told me, 'There is a box at school where we can drop a note about any problems worrying us. Next day we are given an appointment to see a counsellor.'

Parents who suspect that their child may be depressed find it hard to get help. Don't give up! Remember, you may be the only 'voice' your child has – so ask and ask again for whatever help is available. Treatment for children is almost always 'talking treatment' with a counsellor or child psychotherapist. If your child is prescribed medication it is important to work out how this is to be taken during school hours. Teachers are not obliged to give medication, but if they agree to do so they must have clear instructions from the medical practitioner who prescribed it.

There is increasing evidence that schools can promote children's mental health and the government is committed to school-based interventions. In June 2001 guidelines were published 'Promoting Children's Mental Health within Early Years and School Settings', and copies of this document are available, free, from the DfES (ref. 0112/2001).

There are other very helpful contacts to follow up. First port of call is, as always, your family doctor who will rule out medical conditions and who should know about the local resources. You should arm yourself with more facts, so check out www.young minds.org.uk and www.young-voice.org. Also, Childline (0800 1111) is a free 24-hour national helpline offering confidential counselling for any child with a problem. The British Association of Psychotherapists has a child and adolescent diagnostic, assessment and treatment service (telephone 0208 452 9823).

Above all, take the signs seriously if your child, of any age, begins to show symptoms of depression.

Children and depression
- Children of all ages can get depressed.
- Early intervention and help will prevent greater problems later.
- Children are responsive to therapy, both psychoanalytic or CBT (cognitive behavioural therapy).
- CAMHS (child and adolescent mental health services) offer specialist mental health care through psychologists, psychiatrists and community psychiatric nurses.
- Beware if your GP dismisses your concerns as a 'parenting problem' or 'just adolescence'.
- Take any signs seriously if you think your child may be depressed. Don't hesitate!

15

ME
(myalgic encephalomyelitis)

A girl lies in bed all day,
Wishing she could run and play
Her face is white as teardrops fall
Still she can do nothing at all.
(Heather McLean, aged 12)

Doubts about its existence

This is a hidden disability which has had a very bad press, it used to be called 'atypical polio' and was thought to be a physical illness until a group of psychiatrists threw doubt on the matter. Subsequently it was identified with a variety of symptoms and the cause was often considered as emanating from problems within the family, most usually stemming from the mother; there was very little sympathy for the condition. And describing it as 'yuppie flu' did not encourage anyone to take it seriously. Indeed, grave doubts were expressed constantly about its very existence. And in some areas of medicine they still are.

In fact, ME is a chronic and disabling neurological disorder, which causes profound exhaustion, together with muscle pain and often an inability to process words and numbers into a meaningful structure. Other typical symptoms listed in the leaflet available from the Tymes Trust, the longest-running national organization supporting children with ME/chronic fatigue syndrome, are:

- memory loss and poor concentration
- loss of balance, co-ordination and fine motor skills
- difficulty sequencing words and numbers, speaking, thinking and absorbing information
- pain (unresponsive to medication)
- headaches
- nausea
- numbness and pins and needles
- sensitivity to light, sound, smells, touch, certain foods and chemical substances
- bouts of racing pulse and breathlessness
- poor temperature regulation
- muscular weakness
- exhaustion, triggered by even minimal exertion (cognitive or physical)
- temporary hyperactivity – resulting in exhaustion
- mood swings, panic, anxiety or depression resulting from brain malfunction and the distress of misunderstood illness.

All these symptoms are generally worsened by physical or mental activity. So a child making an effort to understand class work will quite likely find that this leads to the condition becoming more severe. Most sufferers find that their symptoms fluctuate from day to day, and this may be one reason why observers are sceptical, since they see that it is possible for the sufferer to do something on one day but not on another. An average bout of the condition can last four years, and relapse is a common occurrence.

The precise cause of ME, sometimes referred to as chronic fatigue syndrome or post-viral fatigue syndrome, is unknown. The evidence points to a number of factors coming together to cause this illness, and these include possible immune system defects, a viral infection, genetic causes, emotional factors, such as trauma or bereavement, which can undermine the immune system, a hereditary suscept-ibility, and allergies. Like most disabilities, ME occurs in various forms of severity and can fluctuate. The way that it begins to show itself can vary from person to person but it typically follows a virus infection, although it can come on gradually.

According to Jane Colby, the Chief Advisor of the Tymes Trust, ME is the most widely misunderstood of all illnesses. She says, 'ME is a soul-destroying illness and children have to learn about it: they must sometimes test the boundaries and learn from the relapse which ensues if they go too far.'

A person developing the symptoms of ME is often disbelieved at first, even by his own family. Certainly there are doctors, teachers and other professionals who need a great deal of convincing about the seriousness of this disability. A five-year independent study carried out by Jane Colby and Dr Elizabeth Dowsett showed that 51 per cent of pupils on long-term sickness absence from school were suffering from ME (*Journal of Chronic Fatigue Syndrome*, 1997). This far exceeded the figures for any other illness; cancer and leukaemia, at 23 per cent, formed the next largest category. Schools, families and communities were found to have clusters of the illness.

The symptoms

The symptoms are often lumped together these days as *chronic fatigue syndrome,* and these words can bring about derision as 'fatigue' is quite wrongly equated with tiredness or the kind of weariness we all experience from time to time. 'My son's teacher said to me, "Aren't all adolescents fatigued?" I couldn't believe how out of touch he is.' The difference for children with ME is that they experience *overwhelming* exhaustion plus an array of disabling symptoms.

Each of the symptoms can bring in its wake different problems. Evelyn said that her son has 'sleep problems'. What this actually means is that his sleep is erratic and he may wake at 2 a.m. and not be able to get back to sleep. Other children may not get to sleep until 2 a.m. When a child falls asleep in the early morning, the problem is getting him up for school on time, and indeed this can make a child worse. Some schools allow a pupil with ME to come in later, but others will insist on punctuality no matter what. 'With superhuman effort we got him there at 9.15, but that wasn't seen as good enough. "If he can manage 9.15, he can manage 8.45." The pressure is always put back on the child.' The Tymes Trust runs day training courses for educational professionals to acquaint them with the needs of a child with ME.

People I was in touch with explained that for them the first signs of ME appeared when they were under an additional amount of strain or stress, which can undermine the immune system and make a person vulnerable to infection. Although ME is not caused by stress, it is a very stress-sensitive illness due to cortisol imbalance in the brain that results from the disease process. Could it sometimes be the result of a reaction to a vaccination? Evelyn thinks that her son has not been robust since his vaccination for measles, following which he has had virus after virus (called 'piggy-back virus') and never seems to throw off one before the other takes hold. Samantha: 'We struggled and struggled to get a diagnosis. We went from pillar to post only to find that from the start our GP had noted in his medical files that he had "Post-viral syndrome". Only nobody told us.'

The shock of finding that your body and mind will not respond in the way you want them to is a terrible moment for any child (or adult). This can exacerbate the lack of concentration, attention and cognition caused by the ME itself and these are all signs to alert parents and teachers as well as the child himself to the condition. Andy told me that from one day to the next he suddenly found that it was no longer possible to achieve the 101 things he was supposed to do each day. At first his parents thought he had a virus and made him rest for a couple of days. Feeling better, he then tried to pick up his 'old' schedule, which is the worst thing anyone with ME can do. It must be very hard on any 11-year-old to find he cannot walk very far, or study, without feeling totally wiped out. Andy and his parents had a long way to go before they could get a diagnosis, or find any guidelines about how he could be helped.

I also heard from parents and children that there are marked stages of the illness. Not to recognize these stages means a great deal of heartache for those who are 'encouraged' to do more than they can at any one time. Once more we find that when there is nothing to see there is often disbelief about a disability, and ME still rates very low on the sympathy stakes. This is in spite of the fact that brain function scans can give us something abnormal to see, but they are not often carried out, due to cost.

Education is an area where parents and teachers often seem to fall out too. A child who is 'a little better' may be knocked backwards if he is given too much to do too soon. A teacher who is truly clued in to this debilitating illness will make sure that a child has the notes he requires, but sending him to the library to get them may be too much for him to do on that day.

The problems for a family of a sufferer of ME are immense and, as we heard earlier from Joan (see page 64), she was accused of being the cause of her child's illness because she kept her child at home seemingly 'for her own reasons'. Indeed, in the questionnaire which Young Action Online sent out, 59 per cent of the families had been told by doctors that their children's illness was caused by psychological problems. Although 5 per cent had undergone psychological treatment their parents reported it either had no effect or made the children worse. However, the result about the efficacy of therapy could be different if it were given by a psychologist, counsellor or therapist who truly understands the limitation of the illness, and if it were entered into in a positive frame of mind by all parties, without any blame attached. Many children with long-term illnesses do get depressed *because* of the illness and welcome psychological help to cope with that aspect.

What can help?

An all-too-frequently asked question is whether ME is a physical or psychological condition? To complicate matters, many of the symptoms which point to depression as the primary source are experienced by sufferers of ME as well: disturbed sleep and feeling slowed down being two of these. As with any illness a person is more at risk if he is under stress, which undermines the function of the immune system. But almost all the experts who understand ME agree that it is not just stress, but a combination of factors which contribute to the severity of the condition. One thing which can muddy the waters is that someone with a history of depression may develop secondary depression or anxiety because of the illness. Not surprisingly this is especially so when there have been disagreements about whether ME is a condition to be taken seriously or not. However, certain aspects of brain chemistry in depression are the *exact opposite* of brain chemistry in ME, showing that the two conditions do not share the same pathology.

There is some evidence that antibiotics may help some people. But as ME is most likely caused by a virus, in many cases it does not help. However, if there is an infection in the body the antibiotics will clear that up, and as a result the ME sufferer will feel marginally better.

Two areas of help have been found beneficial by some families I have spoken with. Cognitive behaviour therapy is one, and graded exercise is another. Neither are cures, but they can be helpful if tailored to meet the requirements of *some* people. Once a programme is agreed on, if it does not proceed steadily due to muscle malfunction, it is demoralizing for all concerned when going even a little too fast brings on a relapse. Great caution must be urged on anyone proceeding down one of these roads. As ME is potentially a relapsing illness it should be kept in mind at all times that putting on the pressure will backfire. Indeed, being able to cope with relapse is one of the hardest nuts to crack. Again, from Jane Colby: 'Doctors have been advised by their medical defence unions that prescriptions for exercise must be given with as much care as those for medication'

(Letter to *Physiotherapy Frontline*, December 2001). So play safe with the healing process.

The best kind of help seems to come from the support of loving family or friends. Your child will need assistance keeping up his spirits, and this is where a parent's attitude is so important in maintaining the right balance. In addition to this, a parent will often have to be a buffer between the child and the outside world where the attitude may be less sympathetic. Beware to of 'goals' – the bane of an ME sufferer's existence. They often serve to cause stress and result in a sense of repeated failure to achieve. 'Pacing' is much safer and is an alternative treatment involving living within one's limits while the body heals. Then the limits slowly expand. Don't aim at anything that is not achievable, and nurse and encourage your child making sure they do not feel forced into some kind of race towards a target.

Helena told me that once she and her daughter had accepted the diagnosis of ME, they began to relax, but then the problems started. Explaining the illness to other people can be very time-consuming; and it is frustrating if you have to convince them about the very existence of the illness. Her advice was, 'Don't waste your time explaining to people who are sceptical, it's not worth it. Spend the time with your kid instead.' She also told me once again that the important thing is to work out strategies with your child to help him cope: 'Play or work for a bit, then stop and rest, whether you are tired or not.' Helena said her worst battles were with the education authorities who, once they could see some improvement, wanted to pile on the pressure for her child to 'catch up'. Jim told me that he thought it very important to keep his son away from anyone who believed that 'Jack could do it if he wanted to', or, 'Just stop him eating the wrong food, and he will be fine.' 'Why', asked Lorraine, 'does everyone think they are an expert on your kid? Within a few weeks we were told (1) to let him stay in bed for a month and (2) to get him out for brisk exercise.'

Alison told me that her daughter began to be very tired – sometimes sleeping for up to seventeen hours. The GP said it was to do with growing up. Jenny began to be very weepy and complained of pains in her legs and lower back. Again, 'She is outgrowing her strength,' from the GP, but Alison requested a referral to a paediatrician. 'They won't find anything,' was the reply. Then endless waiting for an appointment with Jenny complaining of pains in her legs, sensitive to sound, eyes going fuzzy and very tired. The paediatrician suggested antidepressant tablets, but a new GP knew just what was happening. 'I thank God for that day,' said Alison. 'Jenny has been very ill, taken into hospital and at one time, tube-fed. Gradually we have got Jenny back with his help.' Jane Colby and the Tymes Trust have helped Alison and Jenny in their struggle with the education authorities, when too much pressure was put on this child by a tutor.

Protection from overload

Children experience much duress from schools to get back to class, and of course many children are desperate to get their 'old life' back as quickly as possible. As a parent you will find yourself between a rock and a hard place as you try to negotiate between the two. It will be tough going to get across to some teachers that although your child may sometimes be able to make a great effort for a while, they will pay the price later. Of course, there are some schools and teachers who understand very well, and will make sure your child gets the support needed: extra time for any exams, perhaps taking them at home, a short school day, or concentration on only a few subjects instead of the whole syllabus. And not taking any tests that are unnecessary, such as SATS (Standard Assessment Tests – measuring a child's performance in school). A really supportive teacher will find a quiet place for a child to rest, perhaps several times a day. It is important, too, not to let a child feel this is a punishment, and care should be taken so that he does not miss out on good things which are going on at school. Even if your child has not been statemented, it may be necessary to ask for an Individual Education Plan. The best support a child can have is when there is a true parent–teacher partnership.

Brain scans of children with ME show that when effort, physical or mental, is undertaken, blood flow in certain areas of the brain *de*creases and the oxygen supply is reduced. This makes the process of thinking impossible. Research has shown that the ability of people with chronic fatigue syndrome is significantly disrupted, which only proves what people with ME know all too well: that a train of thought can easily be lost.

Parents often have a very hard time when they are trying to protect their child from overload, so be prepared for this. You may even be accused of condoning school absence, or of Munchausen's Syndrome by Proxy; again and again I heard from parents who had been told that their children's illness was due to 'psychological problems'. In 2001 *The Times Education Supplement* Scotland published an article where ME was described as 'Mother's Encouragement' to stay off school. ME, more than any other invisible disability, seemed to carry this stigma. Needless to say, the paper subsequently had to print a good deal of information to the contrary, and an editorial distancing themselves from that statement.

Together with your child you should draw up a list of what makes him feel under pressure thus increasing the fatigue. Take care that he does not feel you are blaming him for 'doing too much' and so making himself ill. We are talking about the over-stress which can bring on a relapse. Learn from each experience. One family told me that they always plan to do things which are a treat, but at the same time prepare themselves to cancel if the moment is just not right. There will always be another day. And small treats can be better than over-demanding ones.

As conventional medicine cannot offer much help, many sufferers turn to complementary medicine. Acupuncture, massage, relaxation, meditation, shiatsu, homeopathy and osteopathy have all been reported to be helpful to some people, together with psychotherapy. Opinions differ about the use of diet, supplements and vitamins. All this points to the need for more research into the cause and treatment of ME. However, it is known that due to disturbed digestion, certain foods will cause pain and bloating, so a modification of diet for a while can relieve these symptoms.

A major teaching hospital in London has a rehabilitation programme based on cognitive behaviour therapy, tailored to each person's individual needs. For Sydney the centre was a lifeline. He was a busy head of school when, in his words, 'I crashed. My GP didn't believe me, but eventually I found out about this research unit.' Clinical and research evidence in those who are *not* severe cases and are ambulant and able to attend a unit regularly support the use of CBT for CFS in those groups of patients, but the information handed out by King's College Hospital warns that 'Neither we nor anyone else claims that CBT is a "cure" for CFS – nor that it works for every person.'

The Tymes Trust also offers support to children and help to parents and doctors, teachers and social workers who can all consult with an ME expert and a fellow professional. Call their advice line (01245 263482) or visit www.youngactiononline.com. The ME Association (www.meassociation.org.uk) has a 'listening ear' service, which is available every day of the year (telephone 01375 361013), where there is always someone to talk to about the illness and its symptoms.

Margaret, the Countess of Mar, wrote an important article in *The Times* (11 July 2001). She believes that one of our most important laws, the Children Act 1989, is being misused to accuse innocent parents of seriously harming their sick children and for social workers (under section 47) to enforce potentially harmful treatment on the children without parental consent. 'The children in question are often severely disabled by an illness for which science has yet to find a cure – ME.' Without evidence, parents are blamed for their children's illness and the child protection law is invoked: 'Sometimes children are taken away from parents and subjected to often futile cognitive-behavioural therapy and physical exercise.'

Information about ME is steadily increasing, but do not get too demoralized if you come up against someone who does not know about this illness, or does not believe it exists. Anyone who has either experienced the debilitating symptoms or watched someone struggling with the uncontrollable ups and downs of this disability knows about the limitations it can impose on a child and his family.

Remember your child needs a life too, so don't hold back on any appropriate social event he feels like attending in the hope it will mean that he can go to school early next morning. The opposite may well be true, and only trial and error will show the way.

The latest Report (January 2002) from the chief medical officer at last gives official recognition of CFS by the Government. The Government-appointed working group has given the first firm guidance to professionals on how to treat and manage ME. This is the reaction of Jane Colby, a member of the Government Working Group that compiled the report: 'No treatment so far developed is a cure and some may even do harm, so it is good practice to encourage the patient to become the expert in self-management. The child and the family may choose how to manage the illness, having considered all the expert advice offered to them.'

And a last word from Jane Colby: 'What is needed is a good old-fashioned convalescence.'

Facts and recommendations about ME

- It is estimated that up to 300,000 people in the UK have ME. Around 25,000 are thought to be children.
- Watch out for your child's frustration. He may be feeling he 'should' be better.
- Do not encourage a child to go on working or studying once symptoms begin to show again. Even better, try to stop symptoms recurring by letting him study in short bursts.
- Remember that travelling to school or just moving around the school building may bring on symptoms, and bring about a relapse. Home tuition or distance learning are good options.
- Keep distractions to a minimum if your child needs to concentrate on work.
- Most people experience gradual improvements over time, but there may be relapses on the way.

- He should not strive to reach the same level of activity as before the onset of ME.
- Be kind to yourself – or your child – if memory and ability are unreliable.
- Many complementary therapies, while not a cure, may help the symptoms.
- Keep a diary to help you pinpoint what causes which symptoms – a delayed reaction is very common.
- Energy management is the only safe known way to assist self-healing.
- Remember: the classic symptom that differentiates ME from other illnesses and forms of fatigue is when the body is unable to recover from physical or mental effort.

16

Tourette syndrome

'She couldn't help herself,' I said. 'She suffered from a neuropsychiatric disorder called Tourette's syndrome. Sometimes it manifests itself as coprolalia which is a compulsion to utter obscenities.'

(Minette Walters, *The Shape of Snakes*)

Signs and effects of the syndrome

This is a chronic neurobiological disorder characterized by both motor and phonic tics. The first case was diagnosed in 1825 by a French doctor, Dr George Gilles de la Tourette. TS is a widely misunderstood neurobiological condition, and as yet there is no cure, although the symptoms do tend to decrease as a child gets older. And if the symptoms are severe, medication may help. According to the Tourette Association over 29,000 people in the UK are diagnosed with this disorder, but this figure is almost certainly an underestimate. Studies conducted independently in the UK and the US agree that 3 per cent of the general school population have enough symptoms for diagnosis of TS although the vast majority may be unaware that this is so (UK: Mason et al., 1998; USA: Kurlan et al., 1994).

TS is a spectrum disorder ranging from very mild to severe. It can begin quite suddenly, and may go hand in hand with other disabilities, especially ADHD, OCD (Obsessive Compulsion Disorder) and ritualistic behaviour (where actions are repeated over and over again, often in a specific order). Like so many other hidden disabilities, it is more common in boys than in girls and the onset is usually between the ages of six and nine. The first signs to alert a parent to this syndrome may be rapidly blinking eyes or facial twitches. The motor tics can occur anywhere in the body but for most people it is the face, head and neck. There are no blood tests or neurological testing which can be called upon to diagnose TS.

Although most of the people with Tourette will not have learning difficulties, they may still have special educational needs. If TS goes hand in hand with another disorder, or if a child has real problems dealing with a specific tic, this will call for educational assistance. For example, timed tests may present a very real problem for a child who is distracted by making sounds or movements.

What causes a major problem for families is that even the most sensitive parents at times cannot believe that the actions are completely involuntary. As well as physical signs, grimacing, twisting around, sniffing, grunting and more, another distressing symptom is uttering words repeatedly, often obscene words. They are often referred to as 'inappropriate' words, and although coprolalia (using inappropriate or unacceptable words or phrases) does not occur in all cases (only 10–15 per cent of cases) it is a symptom often seized upon by the media, and where it is present can cause untold grief to parents and children alike. Lydia was prepared to describe to me in graphic detail what distresses her and her family: 'He spins and he reels while shouting things like, "Up your butt bitch!" and, "Around the corner to your dick . . . oh sorry you haven't even got one." He just goes on and on and is penis-fixated.'

Case histories

The Shaw family thought they had enough to worry about with a boy with severe ADHD, but a phone call from the school complaining about the sexual content of their son's conversations sent them into turmoil. 'I have to shut myself in the bathroom at times because I just can't cope any more with the day-in day-out problems,' said this mother. 'I can't believe he can't help himself, but if ever there is a pause it all comes out in a burst a few hours later, and that is even worse.' 'It will be "invisible", all right,' said another father to me, 'we just won't let him out of the house.'

Brendan told me that his son is a whirling dervish from the moment he wakes at 6 a.m. 'My son has ADHD plus Tourette and until we force the med into him it is a constant stream of potty talk and making so much noise that I forget all the things I have learnt at parenting classes.' Brendan and his wife Charlotte said they were desperate for help and went to parenting classes as they were told. The strategies did not work, and they felt that everything was falling apart. 'Sometimes something seemed to work for a while, and then bang, back to square one.'

Waiting for appointments to see a psychologist or psychiatrist is something that many parents complained of. However, when one mother eventually did get an appointment a consultant child psychiatrist said, ' "Yes, you are right, your son has difficulties." "Difficulties?" I asked, "What does that mean?" The reply was, "Well – he's bright, very bright, easily bored and quite active, but there could be something you are doing wrong. Do you, you know, get down on the floor and play with him?" I was speechless.'

'I have been told by the professionals that it is my attitude to the swearing which causes the problems and *I* need to change.' This mother, too, had taken parenting courses. 'I can't help taking the words personally, the constant use of mother****** just wears me down.'

Do drugs work? Some tics can be minimized by medication, but it is important that they are prescribed by a doctor who has had experience in treating TS. There is no one specific medicine to help a child with TS. Parents reported that their experience was that the medication most frequently prescribed for ADHD often has the effect of increasing the tic movements. Many TS patients prefer to live with the tics rather than take medication. Tranquillizers may be prescribed, but parents complained that they only made their child lethargic on top of everything else. Sometimes antidepressants are prescribed, usually when there are accompanying obsessive compulsive symptoms as well. However, the majority of children with mild TS are not under the care of a doctor.

Andrea: 'I think meds do help. We have just given him a drug holiday, and ohmigod, it is not something I would wish on my own worst enemy.'

Coping with the difficulties

According to a professor of neurology at the University of Rochester Medical Center in the US, Tourette syndrome is really very common, usually with mild symptoms. Somewhat reassuringly he believes that this does not progress to the severe form. While tics, shouting obscenities or jerking are evidence of the syndrome, there are other repetitive and involuntary movements which are often seen as no more than annoying, or nervous habits. Signs like clearing one's throat repeatedly, or rapid eye-blinking. Children who show these signs may be subjected to teasing from other kids and constant fidgeting may get them into trouble at school, but they are not necessarily diagnosed as having TS.

So what is it like to be a child with a tic? Andrew: 'I was called Blinky at school, but I didn't mind. But in my early teens I started to produce the grunting noises – as my parents would lovingly call them. What really hurt the most was that my parents would tell me to stop grunting and to be quiet. It's quite distressing when you can't stop something like this and you are embarrassed to talk about it as well. The first thing you feel is isolation, as the two people you love most in the whole world are getting short of patience with you over something you can't control. With no one to turn to life seems pretty bleak at times.'

'When I first heard of TS from a TV programme it didn't make me feel any better. I'm thinking that in years to come I'm going to be shouting swear words at people and jerking around a lot like the people we saw on TV.'

To suffer from TS is likely to cause emotional problems because of the way people react to the symptoms. Justin told me that he tries to control his movements, but it means that he has to sit in the back row of a theatre or cinema otherwise people complain about his head-jerking movements. Dave told me that because he sniffs all the time, people think he has a cold and he goes along with this to cover his embarrassment. Gordon mentioned that the worst thing for him is that people tell him to stop and be quiet because they think he can stop, but he can't. 'No one is as kind to you as they are to visually disabled people.'

Ben sent me this email: 'I am not diagnosed with TS but I am sure I have it. I have covered it up quite well during my life although on occasions friends might comment on a twitch, and I will just joke it off or say that I am tired. Sometimes it really gets me down and I cry to myself. I have *never* talked to anyone about this.'

It is very hard for a family to cope with the chaos imposed on everyday life by someone with this disorder, who is likely to be impulsive and be easily distracted. As with other disabilities, parents are often confused about how to distinguish between the symptoms of the disability and plain bad behaviour. One helpful way is to talk to another parent of a child with TS. An excellent starting point could be Tourette Syndrome Support – a website hosted by a mother who wanted to provide information about TS in the UK (www.tourettesyndrome.co.uk).

And, of course, any parent who is concerned about their child in this respect should contact the Tourette Syndrome Association. It was founded in 1980 and is an invaluable source of information and support. It also has a very interactive website (www.tsa.org.uk) which enables families to exchange ideas and strategies. The TSA believe that it is important to recognize TS as early as possible, and it acknowledges that parents may be overwhelmed by their child's bizarre behaviour, for which family therapy has been found to be most helpful. Behavioural therapy, relaxation techniques and biofeedback can also all help to alleviate the stress reactions which cause the tics and involuntary movements to increase in frequency.

Some facts about Tourette syndrome
- Tourette syndrome is a spectrum disorder ranging from the very mild to severe.
- The majority of children with Tourette syndrome have it in a mild form.
- As well as Tourette syndrome there may be additional problems such as ADHD, OCD, LD and difficulties with impulse control and sleep problems, the condition known as 'Tourette syndrome plus'.
- The only symptoms are often motor or vocal tics, with no behavioural or educational problems.
- Coprolalia (the use of inappropriate or unacceptable words) occurs in only 10–15 per cent of cases.
- On a more positive note, TS sufferers can be more than usually creative, with acting ability and a talent to mimic.

17

The last word

Parents learn a lot from their children about coping with life.
(Muriel Spark, *The Comforters*)

From the parents

All parents who are worried about their child want to know, 'What is happening to him and *why?*' And this is swiftly followed by '. . . and what can we do?'

When I spoke to those mothers and fathers who devote much of their lives to supporting a child with special needs a contented minority told me that they were blessed to have a special child. They felt they had become kinder and more sensitive to others. Sally even went so far as to say that having a child with severe learning difficulties was a wonderful thing: 'As a family we are more compassionate and loving than we were before my daughter was born.'

Others said they were 'coping' or 'struggling' or 'desperate' and spoke of their grief at the sadness of it all. Of course, there are broken dreams and while other parents worry about drug abuse or sexual promiscuity, parents of a child with special needs have a lot more on their minds. 'Will their child cope at school?' 'Will he be bullied?' 'Will he make friends?' And, 'Will anyone please explain what is happening?' 'Is there anyone who can help my child?' 'Should I try this, or should I try that medication or diet?' And, most pronounced of all, 'What will happen to my child when I can no longer look after him?'

'Grief, GRIEF, GRIEF,' said Tracy. 'The tears I have shed into my pillow would float a battleship. The outside world doesn't know about that. I am a leading light in getting resources – I raise money – I even counsel other parents, but underneath my heart is breaking as I see Jimmy struggle every day.'

'I have two boys who have Asperger and it's hard for me to accept that our genes managed to do this – twice.'

'Unless you have a child with an invisible special need you can have no idea of what it is like to be part of a family caring for such a child. The outside world has no idea, no idea at all.'

Henry, a father, told me that on the surface he seems fine, but underneath there is anger and a continual concern about the future. 'Some of which I manage to block out a lot of the time. But, I feel robbed because some of the things I looked forward to doing with a son are not going to be possible. His language and behavioural difficulties have affected the quality of my relationship with him. I suppose part of me is always seeing the problem and not the person.'

Several parents told me that the best way to proceed was 'to slow down'. What exactly did they mean? They felt that as they become totally involved in the frantic search for a diagnosis, for a cure and for help for their child, there is no time left for anything else. If a child has severe ADHD then the entire family gets caught up in a whirlwind of activity. So 'take stock' is what they advise. The Murray family provide a salutary lesson: 'Two boys with severe ADHD, a daughter with ADD. All our time and energy go in to just *containing* them – we never go on outings or on holiday. We just try and get through each day.'

Several parents told me how they are embarrassed when people say to them, 'Oh, you are wonderful,' or words to the effect that they are saints to care for their child in the way they do. 'We are *not* saints,' said Norman, 'in fact if I tell the truth I hate my boy at times. He causes chaos wherever he goes, makes his sister's life a misery, and my wife has had a nervous breakdown brought on by his behaviour. There, I have said it out loud.' Not many parents were prepared to speak so bluntly, but it wasn't necessary: I saw with my own eyes the strain on the faces of those who have to cope with endless broken nights and fractured days.

'What I can't stand is when people look horrified and full of pity for our situation, but we have never known things to be different. We accept our children for what they are. Some days they are great, but there are terrible days you would like to forget. I never look further than a couple of days at a time.'

The 'terrible twos' are a trying period for all parents, but the temper explosions of a child of nine or older are a nightmare in comparison. Janie and her husband have developed a strategy whereby they try to circumvent any situation likely to build into a scene: 'My child is bright and copes at school. She is on Ritalin, but when she gets home the slightest thing sets off an explosion, the like of which you wouldn't believe. My other kids run for cover.' These parents are quite sure this is not 'giving in' because they believe that as their daughter cannot help the outbursts, she has no control over them. They feel it is their job to make sure as best they can that she is not provoked in any way, and they hold on to the belief that over time her communication skills will improve and the screaming, biting and hitting will decrease. They are already beginning to see a slight improvement, and this gives them the strength to carry on.

In her book *Can't Eat, Won't Eat*, Brenda Legge tells what it is like from a mother's perspective to have a child with Asperger syndrome who won't eat 99.9 per cent of all known foods. Other parents who contributed to her book tell of the tremendous problems of living with a child on such a restricted diet. 'Our little boy is diagnosed as autistic and has an overwhelming fear of change. This includes food, which has to be the same limited diet every day. I feel like screaming sometimes, but then I sit quietly for a moment and remind myself that it is fear of anything new which is behind the apparent stubbornness.'

I have given accounts in earlier chapters of the difficulties of getting a diagnosis but these words from a mother in Australia encompass the dreadful journey for many parents: 'My son was not diagnosed as autistic until he was three and a half, despite constant trips to various specialists from the age of eighteen months. Before we reached that crucial diagnosis Bob had been labelled as ADHD – the ultimate one-size-fits-all diagnosis in this country – and developmentally delayed, deaf (he wore hearing aids unnecessarily for almost three years!) and emotionally disturbed. One doctor suggested I was a touch neurotic, while another bluntly suggested I was simply an inexperienced mother with too much time on her hands.' Cindy Dowling is now using this experience to collaborate with Benny St John Thomas to write a book to be called *So Long As Its Healthy*, a collection of material from parents struggling to come to grips with a child's disability.

A failure to diagnose the real reason for a child's abnormal behaviour can all too easily happen if there are other more obvious causes: 'We adopted a daughter who is now twelve years old. She was born addicted to crack, eight weeks premature, blind in one eye, hearing impaired in one ear, ADHD, learning disabled, and PDD (with a pervasive developmental disorder). Unfortunately, for many years, her obsessive behaviour – thumb-sucking, head-banging, rocking, shyness and many tactile aversions – were attributed to drug exposure and she wasn't diagnosed with PDD until age ten.' This is from Barbara Day who has a website, Guide to Special Education (www.SpecialEd.About.com), so learn from her experience, and if there are several problems for your child make sure that the main cause does not get overlooked or ignored.

From Jody (www.specialchildren.guide@about.com): 'Medication serves a purpose, but unfortunately we often pin our hopes on using medication as a sole cure. This is such a misconception . . . it should be viewed as part of a well-rounded treatment plan that includes reinforcements and behaviour modification.' Jody knows from first-hand experience what she is talking about. She says she has personal guidelines in regard to medicating kids: '(1) I will not medicate a child until first grade in school . . . when the work becomes more difficult. (2) I will not medicate a child with a mild disorder. (3) I will agree to medication, but the dosage should be as small as possible, and (4), if medication produces favourable results, then it's worth it. If I am not seeing positive results in a month, it's time to re-evaluate the situation.'

From a father of a 12-year-old boy with autism: 'Never take "no" for an answer. Apart from a "postcode lottery" regarding resources, the process favours the articulate middle classes. I well remember asking the educational psychologist attached to my son's primary school what happened to parents who could not find their way through the system. Her reply was "they lose out".'

'There is no end to it. I finally agreed to medication for Jamie, but it set off tics. I just don't know what to do next.'

'I gave up looking for a diagnosis. Too much hassle. Every professional we saw said her symptoms pointed to autistic spectrum disorder, *but* she is female and verbal so unlikely. One even told me she was just like an autistic child but can't be because "they all have violent outbursts". Sadly, she is just seen as weird, and because she doesn't understand the games the other kids play they end up teasing her in a very cruel way.'

'Can you explain to other parents and teachers that poor hygiene is sometimes a *symptom* of PDD? Schools don't go along with that one, I can tell you! My daughter Charlotte hates baths, showers and sometimes refuses to change her clothes for days on end.'

'Invisible disabilities? What about FAS (foetal alcohol syndrome, which results from prenatal exposure to alcohol)? I have adopted a daughter with FAS and ADD/ADHD and emotional disabilities. I have found that there is more help for some disabilities than others. Because she is young and pretty I hear from all sides, "She's an attractive young lady, what's wrong with her?" and, "How can anything be wrong, nothing *look*s wrong!"'

What other help would parents like?

This question opened a floodgate from parents, ranging from 'I don't *know* what help I want' and 'Anything, *anything*', to a detailed list of the support parents need. For parents of children with ADHD practical help came high on the list. Most mothers told me that help which was often there when their child was very small, dried up as he became older and more difficult to contain. Anger was expressed at the way help was there before a birth – with antenatal classes and then breast-feeding support – and then nothing. *Nobody wants to know* was the key phrase and from the evidence I was shown this is how it looked.

Those who could afford to pay for help found it hard to find the right kind of person to care for a child even for a few hours a week. Judith: 'We could afford some help a couple of afternoons a week to give me a break and so I could catch up on my sleep. But it soon became obvious that although carers came for an interview and said they understood the problem, and that they were interested to work with a child with special needs, it never lasted very long.' A series of daily helps, au pairs and even a nanny resulted in Judith's son becoming more hyperactive and more difficult to manage.

Almost all parents said they wanted more practical advice and information. Help of any kind is patchy in the UK, and it is almost a lucky dip to expect to find help from your local authority. Some social services offer a respite place in a nursery, perhaps once or twice a week, and this is always seen as a godsend. Wherever you live, all help has to be *searched* for. So, this is an area where other family members can really lend a hand: for instance, retired grandparents may have the time needed to ferret around for practical aid.

Mothers were often desperate to find a support group, and I heard repeatedly of a longing to share experiences with other parents who know what it is all about. To speak to someone who has been there and perhaps found a solution can be like striking gold. Fortunately, the Internet now has a range of websites and interactive chat rooms which are a boon for lonely and worried parents. To be in touch with someone who knows just what you are going through and will be sympathetic to your fears for the future can be reassuring. You may even feel free to express feelings which you are reluctant to share with your partner: for instance, about how often you feel you cannot go on and how you resent the way that your child with special needs has taken over family life. When you hit a rough patch you need encouragement to keep on going, and this can sometimes come more satisfactorily from outside the family.

It is sometimes impossible for a parent to dredge up the extra energy to campaign for more resources. But, if you have the strength, ask your health visitor if she knows how you can make contact with other parents in a similar situation, or put a letter in your local paper. You will be surprised at the response. That was how I came to know many of the parents who have shared their experiences in this book; all those who telephoned me were only too willing to talk about the difficulties they had come up against.

Financial help

It has to be admitted that a lot depends on finance. Often 'poor resources' was the reason given for help not materializing or for waiting lists for appointments being interminable. And all too often help that was on offer dried up because of lack of cash. Wanda said that her little girl is at a nursery school where they are 'wonderful with kids with special needs'. Sadly, this is now the last year that this school will be funded and so it is going to close. The children are to be incorporated into mainstream nursery, but Wanda says that for most of them it will not be suitable. 'It all boils down to money,' she told me.

Parents who at the start could ill afford the consultation fees, felt driven to go on looking for help in the private sector. Families who were told that speech and language therapy, occupational therapy or a special diet might possibly help felt bound to find the money somehow.

The children speak

I heard from many adults who suffered when they were growing up because their handicap was invisible to the outside world. When they were children they *knew* that 'something was up' and that somehow they were not in step with the rest of the world. Steven used the expression 'not clicking in' when he was telling me what it was like to have Asperger syndrome and to have to get along without any acknowledgment or understanding from anyone. He said he used to sit and watch the other children joking around while he fought back tears because he could not understand what was happening. As he got older it became worse for him. Social situations were a nightmare, and he soon found that people in general are not at all tolerant of an adult who shifts around in his seat, takes any everyday phrase or metaphor literally and who always looks uncomfortable in company. Repeatedly he asked himself, 'What's wrong with me?' 'Why don't I fit?' And, 'Why can't I click in?', just as we heard from Clare Sainsbury, who struggled as she grew up to make sense of her own disability. To do this on your own must be a terrible burden.

It is important to remember that ADD/ADHD and Asperger syndrome can persist into adulthood. And some of the most articulate comments came from adults who recalled their experiences as children: 'A diagnosis of autism was not made until I was in college – I had struggled for years and I was told I couldn't be autistic because I was a female and talkative, and had no obvious learning difficulties. I knew I was different, though. Once I grew up I found out all I could about the problem I had with processing information. Meanwhile I was accused of wanting a "syndrome of the week", but at the age of thirty I got my diagnosis. Now I get the help I need.'

'I had undiagnosed ADD for thirty-one years. I got no help, and have very low self-esteem. I just about gave up on everything and got very depressed. I used to ask myself, "Who cares?" and answered, "Nobody".'

'I was diagnosed as having ADHD as a kid. I have lost the "H" as I have got older, but now I just get depressed.'

'I went through hard times including low self-esteem, suicidal thoughts, social phobia and an obvious inability to concentrate or to complete tasks. This has led to constant job-hopping and no personal success. That's what ADD can do to you.'

From June I heard a similar story of struggling to be recognized as having a handicap: 'I suffered all through school and jobs because of some yet-to-be-determined disability. I was/am extremely articulate and spoke intelligently. People thought I was intelligent, bright and a good asset to their social set. However, I found myself not understanding directions clearly, not following instructions carefully, trying so hard and working on projects much too long – and unable to produce the end product. I became overwhelmed and people often got and still get frustrated and angry with me because often my presentation is much better than my product. I can't take tests, and people can't ask me questions because I get flustered and anxious and don't hear the questions clearly, therefore I can't answer correctly. I see the same problems in my son. He doesn't understand simple social situations, personal space, facial cues – things that come second nature to most kids. He just doesn't get it. People do not see our disabilities, they're not physical, they are not "in-your-face-obvious". They are not visible yet many people feel that means you must be fine, and you are just acting and obnoxious. It breaks my heart, because I know my son frustrates and annoys the children in his class.'

'I fell through the cracks at school, and I just sat there quietly. All the help I got was the comment on my report card of "not living up to her potential".'

'I couldn't understand why I missed out on so much. Then my dad talked to me and explained that some people have a certain kind of problem. That helped a lot, and together we think up ways to help me. I carry a bleeper which I set to remind me of things I have to do.'

What is imperative is that the person with a disability should if at all possible recognize it for what it is and work around the condition to find a job and a lifestyle which causes minimum stress. If it is likely that the disability will bring problems with relationships, it is important to be aware of this otherwise the result is likely to be anxiety and depression.

All these 'children' spoke about the loneliness they suffered through their invisible disability. Hopefully, in the future we can ensure that no child is on his or her own with a hidden handicap and that there is help on hand whether the disability is mild or severe.

On medication

'I hated taking Ritalin SO MUCH – I went from feeling full of energy to feeling totally exhausted.'

'The drug I was given always made me tearful and very very tired. The doctor told my mum that it was part of my illness, but I knew it was the drugs.'

'My sister and I were both put on medication, and when we fussed and said it made us feel awful they just increased the dose. I can still remember my sister crying and crying, and now my parents tell us that they put us on an antidepressant as well!'

'They soon took me off Ritalin. I was quiet during the day all right, but I can remember I went wild in the evening. They tried to give me sleeping pills but I can remember to this day my grandfather coming and shouting at my parents for pumping me full of drugs. As far as I can remember they stopped just after that.'

From Mike: 'When I was in elementary school I was consigned to failure by my teachers. They told my parents that I would never amount to much, and that I should be labelled "emotionally impaired". My parents didn't listen, and through their love and support, as well as proper treatment, I have managed to succeed. I am twenty-three, and I have been on Ritalin for fifteen years now. I am healthy and I am doing really well at Stanford. Heck! It basically saved my life.'

'Can I butt in? I was like a zombie on drugs but I figured the side effects were proof that the doctor was right and that I really was depressed. I was prescribed them in the first place by someone who didn't know much about ADD.'

'I was on medication for ADD as a child. When I suffered from abdominal pain and insomnia no one believed me. I think they would now, as it is known there are side effects. Nowadays I just manage my ADD.'

'At the age of thirty I went to see a psychiatrist and I am now on Prozac and Adderall and I am experiencing things that I never have before and I have to say it's as powerful as a person who has been blind for their whole life and can suddenly see.'

'At twenty I am not now diagnosed as ADD and instead I am prescribed antidepressants. They work for me.'

'At the age of forty-seven (Phew!) I found out about ADHD and went to a doctor who prescribed medication. It works for my daughter and two sons as well.'

These words need no comment from me.

Recognizing hidden disabilities

My main purpose in this book has been to concentrate on those disabilities which have been 'discovered' or, at any rate, come to the fore over the last fifty years, but where the impact on the child and the family still seems to be underestimated. There are, of course, other invisible disabilities which I have not covered, such as asthma, diabetes and eczema (to give but three examples) and the reason for this is that there is already a whole literature on them available for those seeking wider knowledge and support.

I have been most concerned with those disabilities over which a question mark still hangs, and where the non-specialist is often left high and dry. Times may be changing, but there is still less understanding and recognition of these than of the other more obvious disorders. Advances in knowledge have created subdivisions of some umbrella disorders. For example, dyslexia (or 'word blindness' as it was once called) is no longer always regarded as the same condition and the diagnosis of dyspraxia may even be made instead. The result is that parents desperately seeking guidance often find themselves hopelessly confused.

They soon get lost in the mist surrounding many of the hidden disabilities. Would you call *petit mal* a hidden disability? Until this debilitating illness is diagnosed and treated with medication, many parents are completely bewildered about what is happening when a child is 'absent' for moments at a time. Fortunately, there are now tests which can show whether a child has *petit mal* or a mild case of ADD.

Is school refusal to be counted as a hidden disability? The underlying disability there may well be anxiety, depression or the result of bullying in class. A child refusing to go to school is at first seen as disobedient and difficult to control and the conclusion often is that it is the fault of lack of discipline on the part of the parents. But it is not as clear-cut as this and an adult with a similar difficulty, one which prevented him from going out of the house, would be diagnosed as having agoraphobia. Irritability and extreme moodiness may also be masking depression.

Parents are usually on the look-out for eating disorders, and most will recognize the signs of anorexia or bulimia, which so often herald the start of a worrying illness. Eating disorders seem to affect a larger proportion of girls, but recently there has been a rise in the number of boys diagnosed as anorexic.

What about the more serious illnesses like multiple sclerosis or muscular dystrophy? Until diagnosed there may be a long struggle to understand what is happening to your child.

A child who is profoundly deaf will be diagnosed and help will be at hand, but there are many children who while not deaf fall victim to the education and medical system because they cannot hear well enough. If this is something you suspect with your own child, you should visit Pam's Website at www.hardofhearing children.com and look at her book *Not Deaf Enough*. She says that her son who has 'dysfunctional hearing, dyspraxia and dysgraphia, discalculia, and dysorganization' has just had ADHD added to his list at age seventeen. 'His biggest "dys" ', she says, 'is "dysedugogia" a name someone made up which stands for the inability of the school system to help special needs children.' Pam maintains that the school system has pushed him and the family right over the edge in refusing to help him get through school. 'They just keep pushing a round peg through a square hole,' she says.

The cardinal point about a hidden disability is that the answers only emerge very slowly, if at all. It takes courage to ask the questions, first to oneself, and later to the professionals. When seeking for help outside, often with great effort, there can be real dismay and agony if there is no crisp answer on tap with a ready-made solution. The hoped-for diagnosis, and treatment, may not be there at all. You may never be able to discover the real cause of a certain disability. But keep in mind that the real value of a diagnosis is that it should bring with it a clear indication of the treatment and help available for your child.

How parents can help themselves

Your child may still be very young, and it may take some time to get a clear picture of whether or not he has a special need. In this situation patience can be a virtue, since children can change very dramatically in those early years. Also, our knowledge and diagnosis of different conditions increases all the time. Consider the latest step forward to test unborn babies for Down syndrome: a non-invasive procedure to check for the presence of a bone in the nose can be made, and so an earlier diagnosis is now possible.

Remember, too, that professionals do not always know it all, and you may have to look further to find one who is experienced with your child's condition. Also, it may take considerable time for any parent or grandparent to adjust to a situation; new words and terms have to be learnt. The pain of realizing that your child is not only struggling now, but will have to contend with some difficulties throughout life, can be totally devastating. The irony is that there are times when a full-blown disability brings with it more help and support than there is for those children who are on the mild end of a disorder. Your child's disability may not appear mild to you – when for instance you see how he is battling with reading skills and needs more time than his peers – but very likely because others assess his condition as mild, he will be left struggling to keep afloat.

Again, we all want our children to be liked by others, but a child with behavioural problems will soon be excluded from events. And the most tolerant parent will have great difficulty in managing a condition which is totally chaotic and disruptive. The necessity 'to be there' all the time for such a child is a task most people would find unendurable, but parents go on and on, every moment of their lives. The pain of caring for a child with a severe special need is never-ending.

All parents of children with a disability are hungry for clear and accurate knowledge, and they often have to wade through unnecessary data to find it. Sophie helps to run a support group for parents. She says that she sees the faces of parents struggling to understand why this has happened to them; how they want the answer to 'straightforward' problems such as overcoming difficulties with talking, reading and behaviour. In fact, these are most complex questions. There are so many varying degrees of any handicap.

Take a look at the website of the Henry Spink Foundation (www.henryspink.org). It is an independent charity created to provide disabled children and their families with a comprehensive and accessible information resource. You will find up-to-date factual information about different treatments, therapists, drugs and centres of excellence. They are not a medical organization and do not make any specific recommendations, but they give families enough information to make informed choices for themselves. They provide information over the phone, by email, mail and fax. If they do not have the information on hand, they will point a parent in the right direction. Check out, too, www.drmyhill.co.uk, a website hosted by a doctor which is full of good advice. It is important that every parent has as much information as possible about their child's condition, and thus knows how to take advantage of any help on offer.

But at the end of the day, make room for your child to blossom in his own way. Keep in mind encouraging stories such as that of Nita Jackson. She was bullied at school for being a 'weirdo', but since finding out she has Asperger syndrome she has developed a new objective in becoming a writer. With one play performed and a book on the way she has been inspired by her belated diagnosis. As with autism, remember that many people who have Asperger syndrome can improve significantly and, with help, become more responsive to others.

The 'disability' must be put to the back of your mind for long periods, and the light from your child *as he is* be allowed to shine through. Remember that although your child may not perform in the standard tests as well as you would like, a child's school experience by no means always determines his future success.

Don't let a label of one of the many disabilities listed in this book prevent you from enjoying your child. Don't let the grief you feel for the loss of the child you hoped to have, obscure the good times. Of course, you may wish with all your heart that things were different, but they are not. Ignore criticism from other people or the unkind way they behave towards you and your child.

Do you remember W. H. Davies' poem which begins 'What is this life if full of care, we have no time to stand and stare'? Make sure you, and your child, have time to do just that. Ensure that you see him as the child you love, not just as a child with a disability. Try to focus on fun whenever you can. It is okay to say your child is frustrating, and that at times you feel you come dangerously close to being defeated by it all. It is okay to acknowledge that you feel your heart is breaking when you cannot persuade your child to make eye contact. Don't expect too much of yourself twenty-four hours a day, seven days a week. If the love and security you give your child is unconditional then that will be appreciated by even the most disabled child, and will provide a strong platform for him to stand on for the rest of his life.

You may have decided that your child does *not* have a hidden disability and that the signs that were worrying you have settled down in proportion. Or you may now understand how although there will be *some* struggles along the way, with help and strategies your child will have the space to grow into a special person in his own right. Some children will never do all the things others do, but some will go on to do great things in their own way and live happy lives. I hope this book will have helped you to take a positive and constructive attitude, and to have an even stronger and louder voice on behalf of your child, when and if it is needed. And above all to accept your child for what he is.

A last word from a mother who has been able to embark on this course: 'He has blossomed into a wonderful child, he's funny, he has friends and family that love him. My child's disability is put on the back burner of life. That's not who he is. It's just a postscript at the end.'

I have spoken with many children who are loving, clever, amusing, bright and at times uncooperative, exasperating and annoying. Some had a hidden disability . . . others did not.

About my website

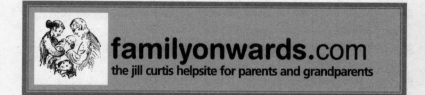

www.familyonwards.com began three years ago as an Internet help site for parents, grandparents and children of divorce. Since then it has expanded to cover many other topics of interest to families.

Responding to the large number of e-mails I receive from men, women and children, the site now includes articles on caring for a child with special needs and reviews of books of particular interest to parents on this subject.

The site also has articles and reviews of books on a wide range of other topics, such as domestic violence, gay family issues, second weddings, marriage, parenting, blended families and many more. New articles, book reviews and notices of videos of interest are posted regularly, and there are links to other helpful and useful Internet sites.

I hope you will visit and contact me on www.familyonwards.com.

Further reading

Allison, Helen Green, *Support for the Bereaved and the Dying in Services for Adults with Autistic Spectrum Disorders*, The National Autistic Society, London, 2001.

Attwood, Tony, *Asperger's Syndrome*, Jessica Kingsley Publishers, London, 1998.

Barkley, Russell A., *Taking Charge of ADHD*, Guildford, New York, 2000.

Breggin, Peter R., *Talking Back To Ritalin*, Perseus Publishing, Cambridge, Massachusetts, 2001.

Cavet, Judith, *People Don't Understand*, National Children's Bureau, UK, 1998.

Clark, Susan, *What Really Works for Kids – the Insider's Guide to Natural Health for Mums and Dads*, Bantam Press, London, 2002.

Colby, Jane, *Zoe's Win*, Dome Vision, Essex, 1999.

Csoti, Marianna, *Social Awareness Skills for Children*, Jessica Kingsley Publishers, London, 2001.

Davis, Bill, *Breaking Autism's Barriers*, Jessica Kingsley Publishers, London, 2001.

Davis, Ronald D., *The Gift of Dyslexia*, Souvenir Press, London, 1995.

Furedi, Frank, *Paranoid Parenting*, Allen Lane, London, 2001.

Hannah, Liz, *Teaching Young Children with Austistic Spectrum Disorders to Learn*, The National Autistic Society, London, 2001.

Hill, Melissa, *The Smart Woman's Guide to Staying at Home*, Vermilion, London, 2001.

Legge, Brenda, *Can't Eat, Won't Eat*, Jessica Kingsley Publishers, London, 2002.

McKay, Pinky, *Parenting by Heart*, Lothian, Australia, 2001.

Sainsbury, Clare, *Martian in the Playground*, The Book Factory, London, 2000.

Smutny, Joan Franklin, *Stand Up for Your Gifted Child*, Free Spirit Publishing, Minneapolis, 2001.

Spungin, Pat and Richardson, Victoria, *The Parentalk Guide to Brothers and Sisters*, Hodder & Stoughton, London, 2002.

Resources

There is now a wealth of information on the Internet, so I have always given web addresses first. Indeed, some of the most useful sources of information only exist as websites and this is why there are no other details for them. Several of the sources are in the United States so you should take care about trying to contact them by telephone or fax.

ADD and ADHD helpline: www.ADDhelpline.org
Adders.org: www.adders.org
Allergy Induced Autism: www.autismmedical.com/welcome.htm
  AiA New Membership: 11 Larklands, Longthorpe, Peterborough
    PE3 6LL
Angels Who Deserve Love:
  http://communities.msn.co.uk/Angelswhodeservelove
Attention Deficit (Hyperactive) Disorder: www.addcontact.org.uk
Body Brushing: www.bodybrushing.com
  PO Box 32, Manchester M24 6SW
  Telephone: 0161 654 4104; fax: 0161 654 4103
  e-mail: steve@bodybrushing.co.uk

Dr Breggin: www.breggin.com/ritalin.html
  Peter R. Breggin, M.D., 4628 Chestnut Street, Bethesda,
    Maryland 20814, USA
  Telephone: (301) 652-5580; fax: (301) 652-5924
British Association of Psychotherapists:
  www.bap-psychotherapy.org
  37 Mapesbury Road, London NW2 4HJ
  Telephone: 020 8452 9823; fax: 020 8452 5182
  e-mail: mail@bap-psychotherapy.org
The British Dyslexia Association: www.bda-dyslexia.org.uk
  98 London Road, Reading RG1 5AU
  Helpline: 0118 966 8271
  Telephone: 0118 966 2677; fax: 0118 935 1927
  e-mail: admin@bda-dyslexia.demon.co.uk or
    info@dyslexiahelp-bda.demon.co.uk
Bullying Online: www.bullying.co.uk
Childline UK: www.childline.org.uk
  Telephone: 0800 1111
Contact a Family: www.cafamily.org.uk
  209–211 City Road, London EC1V 1JN
  Helpline: 0808 808 3555 (freephone for parents and families
    10 a.m.–4 p.m., Mon–Fri)
  Telephone: 020 7608 8700; fax: 020 7608 8701
  minicom: 020 7608 8702
  e-mail: info@cafamily.org.uk
Department for Education and Skills: www.dfee.gov.uk
  Telephone: 0870 000 2288; fax: 01928 79 4248
  e-mail: info@dfes.gsi.gov.uk
The Dyspraxia Foundation: www.dyspraxiafoundation.org.uk
  E-mail: admin@dyspraxiafoundation.org.uk for details of your
    local group or telephone 01462 454986
Exceptional Grandparents:
  http://clubs.yahoo.com/clubs/exceptionalgrandparents
Focus on Disability: www.focusondisability.co.uk

Gifted Monthly Magazine: www.giftedmonthly.com
  The Editor, 28 Wallis Close, London SW11 2BA
  Telephone: 0788 792 3165
  e-mail: info@giftedmonthly.com
Guide to Special Education: www.SpecialEd.About.com
The Henry Spink Foundation: www.henryspink.org
  209–211 City Road, London EC1V 1JN
  Telephone: 020 7608 8789; fax: 020 7608 8790
  e-mail: info@henryspink.org
Home Education Advisory Service: www.heas.org.uk
  PO Box 98, Welwyn Garden City, Herts AL8 6AN
  Telephone/Fax: 01707 371854
  e-mail: admin@heas.org.uk
Homeschooling:
  www.homeschoolyellowpages.com/NFHEE/webrings.html
  24 Windsor Lane, Alpharetta, GA 30004, USA
  Telephone: (770) 664-0960; fax:(603) 368-5878
  e-mail: webmaster@homeschoolyellowpages.com
Hyperactive Children's Support Group: www.hacsg.org.uk
  Sally Bunday, 71 Whyke Lane, Chichester, West Sussex
    P019 2LD
  Telephone: 01243 551313; fax: 01243 552019
The IRLEN Institute: www.irlen.com
Justice Awareness and Basic Support: www.jabs.org.uk
Jabs National Office: Jackie Fletcher, 1 Gawsworth Road, Golborne,
    Warrington WA3 3RF
  Telephone: 01942 713565; fax: 01942 201323
Kingston Special Needs Project:
  www.kingstonspecialneedsproject.org.uk
Learning Disabilities Information: www.ldinfo.com
The ME Association: www.meassociation.org.uk
  4 Top Angel, Buckingham Industrial Park, Buckingham
    MK18 1TH
  Telephone: 01280 818960; fax: 01280 821602
Milton Keynes Support Site: www.mk-adhd.org.uk

National ADD Information and Support Service: www.addiss.co.uk
   ADDISS Resource Centre, 10 Station Road, Mill Hill, London
      NW7 2JU
   Telephone: 020 8906 9068
   e-mail: resources@addiss.co.uk
The National Association for Gifted Children (UK):
   www.nagcbritain.org.uk
   NAGC, Suite 14, Challenge House, Sherwood Drive,
      Bletchley, Bucks MK3 6DP
   Telephone: 0870 7703217; fax: 0870 7703219
   e-mail: amazingchildren@nagcbritain.org.uk
The National Autistic Society: www.nas.org.uk
   393 City Road, London EC1V 1NG
   Telephone: 020 7833 2299; fax: 020 7833 9666
   e-mail: nas@nas.org.uk
Autism Helpline: telephone: 0870 600 8585
   e-mail: autismhelpline@nas.org.uk
The National Deaf Children's Society: www.ndcs.org.uk
   15 Dufferin Street, London EC1Y 8UR
   Information & Helpline: 0808 800 8880
   Telephone: 020 7490 8656; fax: 020 7251 5020
The National Foundation for Gifted and Creative Children:
   www.nfgcc.org
   395 Diamond Hill Road, Warwick, Rhode Island, USA
   Telephone: (401) 738-0937
National Vaccine Information Center: www.909shot.com
   421-E Church St, Vienna, VA 22180, USA
   Telephone: (703) 938-DPT3; fax: (703) 938-5768
   e-mail: info@909shot.com
Parent Partnership Service: www.parentpartnership.org.uk
   8 Wakley Street, London EC1V 7QE
   Telephone: 020 7278 9512
Parenting Support for Unique Families/Adoption and Special
      Needs: www.comeunity.com
Pathological Demand Avoidance Syndrome Contact Group:
   www.pdacontact.org.uk

Raising Kids: www.raisingkids.co.uk

The Royal National Institute for the Blind: www.rnib.com
   Telephone: 0845 766 9999; fax: 020 7388 2034

Smilechild: www.smilechild.com

Special Child: http://specialchild.com/diagnosis.html

Special Children: http://specialchildren.about.com/mbody.htm

Special Families Guide: www.specialfamilies.com

Special Needs Kids: http://specialneedskids.com

Special Needs Project: www.specialneeds.com
   324 State Street, Suite H, Santa Barbara, CA 93101, USA
   Telephone: (805) 962-8087 and (800) 333-6867
   e-mail: books@specialneeds.com

Dr Stordy: www.drstordy.com

Tiger Child: www.tigerchild.com

Tourette Syndrome Association: www.tsa.org.uk
   PO Box 26149, Dunfermline KY12 9WT
   Telephone/Fax: 0845 4581 252 (24-hour voicemail)

Tourette Syndrome Support: www.tourettesyndrome.co.uk

The Tymes Trust: www.youngactiononline.com
   Telephone: 01245 401080

Young Action Online / Tymes Trust, PO Box 4347, Stock,
   Ingatestone CM4 9TE

UKParents: www.ukmums.co.uk

What About the Children: www.whataboutthechildren.org.uk
   60 Bridge Street, Pershore, Worcestershire WR10 1A
   Telephone/fax: 01386 561635

YoungMinds: www.youngminds.org.uk
   102–108 Clerkenwell Road, London EC1M 5SA
   Telephone: 020 7336 8445; fax: 020 7336 8446

Young Voice: www.young-voice.org
   12 Bridge Gardens, East Molesey, Surrey KT8 9HU
   Fax: 020 8979 2952

Index